Also Available From the American Academy of Pediatrics

ADHD: What Every Parent Needs to Know

Allergies and Asthma: What Every Parent Needs to Know

Autism Spectrum Disorders: What Every Parent Needs to Know

Building Resilience in Children and Teens: Giving Kids Roots and Wings

Caring for Your Baby and Young Child: Birth to Age 5*

Food Fights: Winning the Nutritional Challenges of Parenthood
Armed With Insight, Humor, and a Bottle of Ketchup

My Child Is Sick! Expert Advice for Managing Common
Illnesses and Injuries

Nutrition: What Every Parent Needs to Know

The Picky Eater Project: 6 Weeks to Happier, Healthier Family Mealtimes

Raising Kids to Thrive: Balancing Love With Expectations
and Protection With Trust

Retro Toddler: More Than 100 Old-School Activities to Boost Development

Sleep: What Every Parent Needs to Know

Sports Success R$_x$! Your Child's Prescription for the Best Experience

**For additional parenting resources, visit the HealthyChildren bookstore at
shop.aap.org/for-parents.**

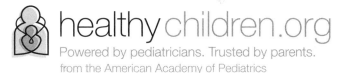

*This book is also available in Spanish.

Achieving a **Healthy Weight** for Your Child

An Action Plan for Families

Sandra G. Hassink, MD, MS, FAAP

American Academy of Pediatrics

DEDICATED TO THE HEALTH OF ALL CHILDREN®

American Academy of Pediatrics Publishing Staff
Mark Grimes, *Vice President, Publishing*
Kathryn Sparks, *Manager, Consumer Publishing*
Holly Kaminski, *Editor, Consumer Publishing*
Shannan Martin, *Production Manager, Consumer Publications*
Jason Crase, *Manager, Editorial Services*
Linda Diamond, *Manager, Art Direction and Production*
Mary Lou White, *Chief Product and Services Officer/SVP, Membership, Marketing, and Publishing*
Sara Hoerdeman, *Marketing Manager, Consumer Products*

Published by the American Academy of Pediatrics
345 Park Blvd
Itasca, IL 60143
Telephone: 847/434-4000
Facsimile: 847/434-8000
www.aap.org

The American Academy of Pediatrics is an organization of 66,000 primary care pediatricians, pediatric medical subspecialists, and pediatric surgical specialists dedicated to the health, safety, and well-being of infants, children, adolescents, and young adults.

The information contained in this publication should not be used as a substitute for the medical care and advice of your pediatrician. There may be variations in treatment that your pediatrician may recommend based on individual facts and circumstances.

Statements and opinions expressed are those of the author and not necessarily those of the American Academy of Pediatrics.

Products and Web sites are mentioned for informational purposes only and do not imply an endorsement by the American Academy of Pediatrics (AAP). The AAP is not responsible for the content of external resources. Information was current at the time of publication.

Brand names are furnished for identification purposes only. No endorsement of the manufacturers or products mentioned is implied.

The publishers have made every effort to trace the copyright holders for borrowed materials. If they have inadvertently overlooked any, they will be pleased to make the necessary arrangements at the first opportunity.

This publication has been developed by the American Academy of Pediatrics. The contributors are expert authorities in the field of pediatrics. No commercial involvement of any kind has been solicited or accepted in development of the content of this publication. Disclosures: The author reports no disclosures.

Every effort is made to keep *Achieving a Healthy Weight for Your Child: An Action Plan for Families* consistent with the most recent advice and information available from the American Academy of Pediatrics.

Special discounts are available for bulk purchases of this publication. E-mail our Special Sales Department at aapsales@aap.org for more information.

Printed in the United States of America
9-396   1 2 3 4 5 6 7 8 9 10
CB0103
ISBN: 978-1-61002-154-8
eBook: 978-1-61002-155-5
EPUB: 978-1-61002-156-2
Cover design by R. Scott Rattray
Book design by Linda Diamond
Library of Congress Control Number: 2017941931

What People Are Saying

Dr Sandy Hassink is one of the most thoughtful clinicians of our time. She has led the fight to ease the epidemic of childhood obesity. Her insights and knowledge are easily communicated in this book written to help parents understand the factors at play and their roles in helping children to live healthier, happier lives. This is a must read for parents, other adults who are in children's lives, and pediatricians. The book is mindful, intentional, and empowering.

Diane J. Abatemarco, PhD, MSW
Associate Professor of Obstetrics, Gynecology and Pediatrics; Vice Chair of Research; and Director of Maternal Addiction Treatment, Education and Research, Department of Obstetrics & Gynecology, Sidney Kimmel Medical College, Thomas Jefferson University

———

This is an honest and open book for parents about how to tackle an epidemic problem: childhood obesity. Dr Hassink draws from her world-renowned expertise to write an easy, readable book that helps parents find simple ways to modify their lifestyles and make sure their kids have a healthy future. I'm excited about this book, especially knowing what insightful information Dr Hassink brings to the table. I hope any parent who is focused on health and nutrition for their child reads this!

Hansa Bhargava, MD
Senior Medical Director, WebMD

———

Dr Hassink is a terrific clinician highly experienced in treating families with obesity. *Achieving a Healthy Weight for Your Child: An Action Plan for Families* reflects her experience and provides practical age-specific advice for families concerned about their child's weight and struggling to do the right thing.

William H. Dietz, MD, PhD
Chair, Summer M. Redstone Global Center for Prevention and Wellness, George Washington University

Parents are their child's first and most influential role model,
protector, teacher, and cheerleader. With this book, Dr Hassink draws
on her years of experience to provide parents with the knowledge they
need and practical tools they can use to actively improve their child's and
family's health. Parents are empowered to reframe nutrition and activity
choices as health decisions, embrace becoming agents of change, and
sensibly address challenges along the journey to raise healthy kids!

Sarah Hampl, MD, FAAP
General Pediatrician and Professor of Pediatrics, Children's Mercy Kansas
City Center for Children's Healthy Lifestyles & Nutrition, University of
Missouri-Kansas City School of Medicine

Dr Hassink is uniquely suited to be the spokesperson for a
comprehensive approach to overweight and obesity. This book
can be used as a reference, or it may be read cover to cover with
many helpful tips for caretakers of children and teens.

Daniel J. Levy, MD, FAAP

Contributors/Reviewers

Author
Sandra G. Hassink, MD, MS, FAAP
Director, AAP Institute for Healthy Childhood Weight

Reviewers
Christopher F. Bolling, MD, FAAP
William J. Cochran, MD, FAAP
Arthur Lavin, MD, FAAP
Gerri L. Mattson, MD, MSPH, FAAP
Joan Younger Meek, MD, MS, RD, FAAP, FABM, IBCLC
Natalie Digate Muth, MD, MPH, RDN, FAAP
Blaise A. Nemeth, MD, MS, FAAP
Tori Smith, parent and advocate
Beth Westbrook Starnes
Yovanni N. Young, community organizer and advocate
for children with special needs

Staff Members
Debra Burrowes
Stephanie Domain
Anjie Emanuel
Sunnah Kim
Ngozi Onyema-Melton
Mala Thapar

To my husband, Bill, and my children and their spouses,
Matthew, Gaby, Stephen, Traci, and Alexa,
for your love, support, and inspiration, and for all
the children and families who struggle daily
to live healthier lives

Contents

Please Note

The information and advice in this book apply equally to children of both sexes, except where noted. To indicate this, we have chosen to alternate between masculine and feminine pronouns by chapter throughout the book.

The American Academy of Pediatrics recognizes the diversity of lifestyles and family arrangements. Please note that this advice applies equally to parents, single-parent families, partners, spouses, grandparents, and others involved in caring for children and adolescents.

The information contained in this book is intended to complement, not substitute for the advice of your child's pediatrician. Before starting any medical treatment or program, you should consult with your pediatrician, who can discuss your child's individual needs and counsel you about symptoms and treatment. If you have any questions about how the information in this book applies to your child, speak to your pediatrician.

This book has been developed by the American Academy of Pediatrics. The authors, editors, and contributors are expert authorities in the field of pediatrics. No commercial involvement of any kind has been solicited or accepted in the development of the content of this publication.

Acknowledgments

I would like to gratefully acknowledge the unfailing help and support of my colleagues who have worked to care for children with obesity and their families over the years in the Weight Management Clinic for Children at Nemours/Alfred I. duPont Hospital for Children in Wilmington, DE, as well as the many colleagues across the country who have dedicated their careers to responding to the obesity epidemic. I would also like to thank the children and families I have cared for, for providing moments of joy, sharing, and inspiration as they journey toward better health.

Introduction

Are you one of the millions of parents who worry about their children's weight? You may have noticed that your child seems to be gaining weight at a faster rate than children of the same age. You might have worried about your family's history of heart disease and type 2 diabetes and wondered if there was a way to protect your teen. Maybe you have felt helpless as you tried to improve your child's and family's nutrition or amount of activity or screen time. Or sadly, you may have anguished when your child came home from school in tears after being taunted and teased because of her weight.

If your child is *overweight* or has *obesity* (see Definitions box), she may be paying the price for consuming large portions at meals or snacking excessively on high-calorie foods. She may be spending too many hours in front of the television (TV) set and not enough time on the playground or soccer field.

DEFINITIONS

Body mass index (BMI): A calculation used by pediatricians using a child's weight relative to height as an initial step to evaluate their weight status.

Overweight: A BMI between the 85th and 95th percentile for age and gender.

Obesity: A BMI above the 95th percentile for age and gender.

Whatever the reason, many parents have a lot of questions about what to do to help their children achieve a healthy weight and are often willing to try just about anything. They might have pleaded with their children to "go outdoors and play" or stop eating unhealthy snacks. They might have tried fad diets or a weight-loss summer camp but with not much to show for it in the long run except frustration.

You Can Succeed!

If you've ever gone on a diet and increased exercise yourself, you know how hard it is to achieve a healthy weight. Being overweight or having obesity is no less challenging for children. The statistics about the problem of obesity in children, which we'll review in Chapter 1, can seem daunting.

Even so, the message of this book is simple: *You and your child can succeed.*

No, we're certainly not going to tell you that it will be easy. You probably know better than that. You and your child may have already done your best to attack the problem for months or maybe even years, and at this point, you may feel very discouraged. You could be thinking that your child is living an ordinary life and that her weight shouldn't be a problem. You may have asked yourself, "She's doing the same things as other kids, so why is she gaining weight?"

In this book, we're going to answer that question and many others and give you the information and skills to help your child adopt good nutrition and activity habits to achieve a healthy weight. We'll start by describing the concept behind this book, setting the stage for what follows.

You Are Not Alone

Parents often feel guilty and blame themselves for their children's extra weight. But obesity is a problem that's bigger than one child, one parent, or one family. In the midst of our thinness-obsessed culture, there is a crisis of obesity in the United States and perhaps in your own home. It affects people of all ages. Ask your pediatrician and you'll probably hear that there has been a dramatic increase not only in the number of heavier children seen in the practice but also in the diseases associated with obesity, including type 2 diabetes and hypertension.

Clearly, there is no need for you or your child to feel isolated in your struggle with this problem. You are not alone. True, your child may feel somewhat "different" because she weighs more than many of her schoolmates. But there are a lot of factors that contribute to your child's weight problems that are making it hard to decide what to do about them.

If it were just a matter of trying to eat less and exercise more, there would probably be far fewer children who have obesity. But with increasing frequency, our society appears to discourage the type of lifestyle that could contribute to normalizing weight. Some schools have cut back or even eliminated physical education programs. Too often, school vending machines are brimming with snack foods like candy, chips, and sugary drinks rather than apples, oranges, and water. Children are spending more time indoors playing computer and video games instead of being physically active. And among parents, jam-packed schedules are forcing many of them to reduce their meal preparation time, which often results in greater reliance on convenience foods with higher sugar, fat, and sodium content.

It's a Family Issue

Obesity tends to run in families. Your child is much more likely to have obesity if you or your spouse (or your child's grandparents) do as well.

Even so, you shouldn't blame yourself for your child's weight problems. Don't blame your spouse or your child, either. Yes, perhaps your child is a little too sedentary, or maybe she's eating too much, but there's no malicious intent on anyone's part. The blame game is just going to get in the way of helping your child succeed, once and for all.

At the same time, you need to be aware that there are many ways in which you and other family members can start contributing to your child's success in achieving a healthy weight. Family attitudes, dynamics, and behaviors are powerful influences on your child's willingness to make healthier food choices and increase her physical activity. Remember that your family is on this journey *with* your child and the support you get from each other can be one of the most important ingredients in achieving a healthy lifestyle. For example

- Children watch what you do. Telling your child what to eat and how much to exercise is not enough; you need to become a role model for healthy eating and activity.
- Helping your child make good decisions about eating and being active in ways that are supportive, and not critical, is crucial.
- High-calorie foods, snacks, and sugary drinks can sabotage healthy eating efforts. Keeping only those foods in the house that fit into your child's nutritional plan is an important strategy for better nutrition.
- Recognizing whether your household uses food as comfort or your child's weight has become a source of conflict between you and your child helps you take a more effective approach.
- Family meals are important, and eating meals together as a family whenever possible, away from the TV, helps to foster healthy eating habits, especially if your child sees you enjoying the healthy food you have served.
- Screen time can take over a child's schedule; helping your child and family find healthy alternatives to screen time, along with making a screen time routine, can help move the family in a healthier direction.

To help your child succeed, you also need to be realistic about her weight. In some cases, parents may deny that a problem exists. They may believe that their child needs plenty of calories to just grow normally. Or they may tell their pediatrician that they're not concerned about their child's weight, explaining that "everyone in our family is big-boned" or that they're only "a tad on the heavy side." But the first step is facing up to the fact that obesity exists.

The Journey to Weight Loss

Scan the diet books in your neighborhood or online bookstore and you'll see that most promise a quick fix for the problem of obesity. However, these claims of fast and easy changes just don't ring true. In fact, there is a common thread that ties most of these books together—namely, almost none of them work, at least not in the long term.

In this book, however, you won't find promises of instant results. That's just not realistic. Instead, we encourage you and your child to view achieving a healthy weight as a journey. If your child has 20, 30, or 50 pounds to lose, it's not going to happen overnight. *In fact, your best chances of success are to aim for small, incremental changes in her weight-related behaviors over the long term. These small but consistent steps are the foundation on which success can be built, and they're more likely to be sustained over time.*

Think of this journey as taking a walk along a lengthy path and making gradual progress toward your destination, day by day. Yes, like every other road on which we travel, there may be occasional bumps, obstacles, and detours along the way. Almost inevitably, your child will backslide from time to time—maybe she'll binge at a party or splurge on a handful of candy bars at the neighborhood mini-mart. But the key is that the road to weight loss isn't an all-or-nothing proposition. After a setback, encourage your child to be forgiving of herself and get back on the path, headed in the right direction.

Also, remind your child that she is not alone on this journey. You, the rest of the family, and your pediatrician are there to walk with her. It's important for the entire family to be committed to this mission. You can't tell one of your children that "these cookies are not for you—they're for the rest of the family that doesn't need to lose weight" and expect success. The entire family needs to be united, and you and every other family member should be there to support your child every step of the way.

How to Use This Book

In the chapters that follow, you'll find the tools for building a strong foundation that supports a healthy weight for your child. We want you to interact with the content of this book, answering the questions to determine where your child (and family) stands and trying the changes we recommend. This book will be an invaluable companion as your child travels the path toward a healthy weight. Not only will you be able to identify your destination, but you'll also understand exactly how you're going to get there, the checkpoints along the way, the twists and turns in the road you'll be traveling, and how to help your child stay motivated along the way.

As you'll discover, some of the key components involve your child's nutrition and physical activity. *The goal is for her to burn more calories than she consumes.* Much of the book will also be devoted to parenting issues. For example

- In Chapter 2, you'll find sensible nutritional information and guide-lines emphasizing balanced and nourishing meals. We'll stress a diet incorporating a variety of healthful and tasty foods. Again, you won't find a fad diet here; nor will your child feel deprived. As a parent, you won't be asked to count calories or fat grams but only to make and help your child choose healthier foods that can produce changes in her weight. You'll be encouraged to make sure she consumes essential nutrients—protein, carbohydrates, fats, fiber, vitamins, and minerals.
- In Chapter 3, we'll describe the importance of encouraging your child to become more physically active. These days, the average child is less active—and heavier—than children of any previous generation. Children are often over-scheduled with homework, tutoring, and music lessons, and, thus, exercise may be all but forgotten. At the same time, many children watch too much television (an average of almost 3 hours a day). That needs to change to achieve a healthy weight.

- Chapters 4, 5, and 6 will concentrate on important parenting matters relative to childhood obesity and effective weight management. These chapters are key components of this book. As important as proper nutrition and physical activity are, the chances of their long-term success are limited without the sound parenting skills that we'll describe in these chapters. We'll empower you to help your child make changes that can effectively reduce her weight. You'll evaluate how food is used in your family (eg, as rewards or bribes). You'll learn how to partner with your pediatrician, extended family members, and community resources (including grandparents, schools, babysitters, and child care workers) to help ensure your child's success. And you'll learn to deal effectively with a variety of parenting challenges, from your child's emotional turmoil and weakened self-esteem to managing her weight-loss setbacks or detours that will occur from time to time.

In the later chapters of the book (beginning with Chapter 7), we'll describe the developmental stages that all children move through and the way that obesity can affect a child at every point in her life, from infancy and the toddler years to school age and adolescence. At each stage, you and your child will be encouraged to set short-term, achievable goals. Remember, we're talking about changes that will not only help your child manage her weight today but could also keep a serious chronic illness related to her weight from developing in adulthood. Modeling and motivating proper eating and activity today will serve her well for the rest of her life.

Chapter 1
The Problem of Obesity

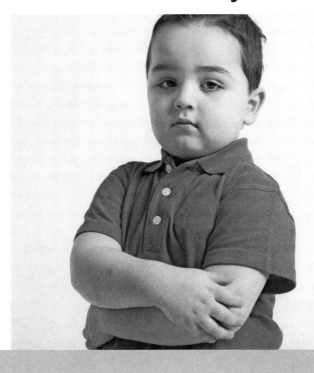

If you spend a few minutes watching children getting off a school bus, you might be surprised by what you see. Amid the expected sights and sounds of kids talking, laughing, and toting backpacks to class, you'll probably also notice a significant number of children who are overweight or have obesity.

In fact, in every corner of the United States—from California to New York and everywhere in-between—obesity among children is at epidemic levels. Just consider the following statistics:

- Since 1980, the prevalence of obesity in children has tripled.
- Seventeen percent (12.7 million) of children and adolescents in the United States have obesity.
- The prevalence of obesity increases with age, with 8.9% of children aged 2 to 5 years, 17.5% of children aged 6 to 11 years, and 20.5% of adolescents aged 12 to 19 years having obesity.

These unsettling trends affect boys and girls. They involve children of all races, all ethnic groups, and all socioeconomic classes. If your child is one of the children affected by obesity, this book offers a way to begin helping him. Whether you have just realized your child has a problem with his weight or have been aware of it for a long time, this book, along with guidance from your pediatrician, can help you and your child find a path through the risks and problems associated with childhood obesity to a healthier lifestyle and a healthy weight. Throughout the rest of this chapter we will be discussing the medical and psychological issues associated with obesity and some common misconceptions that may be getting in the way of moving forward.

The Physical Toll: Medical Diseases and Conditions

Pediatricians are very concerned for many reasons about the growing number of children who have obesity. Not surprisingly, having obesity can limit a child's physical activity on the playground and athletic field. But more worrisome, there are many health risks associated with being too heavy. For example, one study stated that among children who have obesity, 40% already had 2 risk factors for cardiovascular disease, such as high cholesterol levels, high triglyceride levels (another type of blood fat), and high blood pressure. Cardiovascular-related conditions aren't the only health problems associated with childhood obesity (see Your Child With Obesity and the Risk of Disease box).

Diabetes, for example, is another increasing concern among pediatricians and parents of children with obesity. That's because a fast-growing number of newly diagnosed cases of childhood diabetes are the so-called type 2 form of the disease. Type 2 diabetes used to be called "adult onset" because it almost always affected adults, but now this form of diabetes is increasingly evolving into a disease of children and teenagers, as well. In fact, research has shown that about 1 in 3 cases of newly diagnosed diabetes in children are now type 2. Particularly if your child has obesity and is inactive, he has an increased risk of developing type 2 diabetes, and this can mean a lifetime of chronic illness and medication use and result in serious complications, such as loss of vision and kidney function, as well as increased risk of heart disease.

To make matters worse, if your child has obesity, he is much more likely to have obesity as an adult. The statistics are worrisome—about one-third of preschoolers with obesity will grow up to become adults with obesity. That figure rises to about 50% of school-aged children and 80% among teenagers who have obesity. And once your child is an adult, he'll be more likely to have obesity-related health problems, from high blood pressure to joint problems, as well as a greater risk of death, as his weight increases. The bottom line is that obesity can cause a lifetime of very serious health concerns.

YOUR CHILD WITH OBESITY AND THE RISK OF DISEASE

If you child or adolescent has obesity, he has a higher chance of having a number of serious medical problems, including

- High blood pressure (hypertension)
- Abnormal lipid levels
- Type 2 diabetes (once called adult-onset diabetes)
- Asthma
- Sleep apnea (repeated disruption of normal breathing during sleep)
- Skin infections (eg, fungi trapped in folds of skin)
- Pain in the knee, thigh, and hip (often associated with a condition called *slipped capital femoral epiphysis*)
- Back pain
- Liver disease
- Gallstones
- Menstrual abnormalities (eg, irregular or missed periods, known as *polycystic ovary syndrome*)
- Severe headaches with visual disturbances

Disordered Eating

One other point is important to make: Some children become so obsessed with their excess pounds and have such a distorted body image that they begin to try unusual diets, skip meals, or eliminate food groups, further adding to unhealthy eating and poor nutrition. Rarely, some children can become so focused on their weight and body image that they may develop eating disorders, such as bulimia and anorexia, all because they're trying to get their weight under control in an unhealthy way.

Mental Health Concerns

It is important to know that mental health concerns can be increased in children with obesity. Children with obesity have been found to have higher rates of attention-deficit/hyperactivity disorder, conduct disorder, and depression than children without obesity. There are also higher rates of anxiety and mood disorders found in children with obesity who attend weight management clinics. Many children and adolescents with obesity experience bullying and teasing, and this is associated with lower self-esteem and, in adolescents, has also been linked to disordered eating and severe depression. Children with obesity and their parents report lower quality of life, scoring lower on physical and social functioning than children who do not have obesity. Children with obesity may have increased problems in schools, such as increased absences, repeating a grade, and behavior problems.

ENVIRONMENTAL FACTORS

Your child's day-to-day environment—at home, at school, at friends' homes, and virtually everywhere else he spends time—can affect his risk of becoming and remaining overweight. The fast-food restaurants where he eats, television (TV) he watches, and video games he plays can contribute to his likelihood of developing obesity.

For example, the risk of having obesity is more than 4½ times greater for children who watch more than 5 hours of TV a day, compared with children who watch no more than 2 hours a day. That's because children are not only inactive while watching TV, but they also tend to snack at the same time, often eating high-fat foods like cookies or potato chips rather than an apple or a pear, all while watching endless advertisements for high-calorie fast food and sugary drinks. Even so, except for sleeping, most US children spend more time (outside of school hours) watching TV than participating in any other activity.

The Emotional Toll

For children with obesity, as well as their parents, living with excess pounds can be heartbreaking. In its own way, the social stigma attached to having obesity can be as damaging to a child as the physical diseases and conditions that accompany obesity. You can probably see it in the eyes and hear it in the words of your own child. In a society that puts a premium on thinness, studies show that children as young as 6 years may associate negative stereotypes with excess weight and believe that a heavy child is simply less likable.

True, some children are very popular with their classmates, feel good about themselves, and have plenty of self-confidence. But in general, if your child has obesity he is more likely to have low self-esteem than his thinner peers. His weak self-esteem can translate into feelings of shame about his body, and his lack of self-confidence can lead to poorer academic performance at school. The AAP policy statement, "Stigma Experienced by Children and Adolescents With Obesity," provides more information for pediatricians, families, and policy makers on weight bias. For more information on self-esteem and bullying during the school-age and adolescent years, refer to chapters 11 and 12.

You probably don't need a detailed description of how difficult the day-to-day life of children with obesity can sometimes be. They may be told by classmates (and even adults) that being heavy is their own fault. They might be called names and be subjected to teasing and bullying. Their former friends may avoid them, and they may also have trouble making new friends. They could be the last ones chosen when teams are selected in physical education classes.

With all this turmoil in a child's life, he may feel as though he doesn't belong or fit in anywhere. He may see himself as different and an outcast. He'll often feel lonely and is less likely than his peers to describe himself as popular or cool. And when this scenario becomes ingrained as part of his life—month after month, year after year—he can become sad and clinically depressed and withdraw into himself.

In an ironic twist, some children might seek emotional comfort in food, adding even more calories to their plates at the same time that their pediatrician and parents are urging them to eat less. Add to that the other emotional peaks and valleys of life, including the stress of moving to a new community, difficulties in school, the death of a parent, or a divorce, and some children routinely turn to food in times of stress.

There are other obesity-related repercussions that continue well into adolescence and beyond. Teenagers and adults with obesity might face discrimination based solely on their weight. Some research suggests that they are less likely to be accepted for admission by a prestigious university. They may also have a reduced chance of landing good jobs than their thinner peers. Women with obesity have been found to have a decreased likelihood of dating or finding a marriage partner. In short, when heavy children become heavy adults, they tend to earn less money and marry less often than their friends who are of average weight.

GENETICS

The following statistics are for young children and indicate the importance of genetics and family lifestyle in a child's risk of developing obesity:

- ▶ If one parent has obesity a child has a 3-fold greater risk of developing obesity than a child whose parents are both of average weight.

- ▶ If both parents have obesity the child's risk rises by more than 10-fold.

- ▶ For a child younger than 3 years, the presence of obesity in his parents is a stronger predictor of whether he will develop obesity in adulthood than his own current weight.

Childhood Obesity: What Are the Common Misconceptions?

Everyone, it seems, has an opinion about obesity. Some may insist that they know what causes it. Or they might have a dozen or more suggestions on how to conquer it. Yet even though it seems that our culture is obsessed with diets and a belief that you can never be too thin, there are more than enough myths and misunderstandings about childhood weight to go around. Unfortunately, some of this misinformation can get in the way of your child succeeding in his own weight-loss efforts.

To help you and your child get on the right path toward normalizing his weight, let's separate fiction from facts. See if you believe in any of the following misconceptions, and then read what the truth about them is:

"My child and I deserve the blame for his weight problem." Not true. Thanks to the media and many high-profile diet gurus, many children and adults believe that obesity occurs in people who are self-indulgent or weak-willed. With those kinds of attitudes so prevalent, no wonder there's so little empathy and support for individuals who need to lose weight. The fact is that children gain excess weight for a variety of reasons. Some tend to develop obesity because it runs in their families. Others may not make the best selections of foods or portion sizes, often because healthier choices aren't available or perhaps because their parents or grandparents put too much food on their plates. Some children live in communities where it is hard to get enough healthy food. Throughout this book, you'll find descriptions of other culprits and contributors to your child's weight problem that should remove self-blame. Once you understand the causes of obesity a little better, you and your child will be able to manage his obesity more effectively and realistically.

"My child's weight problem needs a quick fix." Yes, you and your child may wish for an instantaneous solution for losing his excess pounds, and there are plenty of diets in bookstores that promise fast results. But let's face it—there are no instant cures to weight problems (or to most other things in life), but there are answers, as you will see in this book. Obesity is not a problem that can be resolved overnight or even in a few weeks. (If you've ever tried to lose weight yourself and keep it off, you know that's the case.) In fact, some of the most popular quick fixes, from diet pills to herbal teas, may be hazardous to your child's health. Many of the "natural" supplements that teenagers might be attracted to, as well as the near-starvation diets that are promoted in newspaper ads and popular magazine articles, are risky and, in some cases, even potentially deadly. Where should you turn instead? Working with your child's pediatrician and using plans and programs, like the one in this book, that are based on credible, scientific evidence offers the best chance for safe and long-term weight-loss success.

"My child will 'grow into' the excess pounds that he has." Some parents tell their pediatricians that their child will outgrow their weight problems. However, that's not something you can count on. In fact, depending on your child's eating habits and activity level, he is just as likely to continue to gain weight, and not lose it, as he grows. Don't depend on routine growth spurts to compensate for his weight problem.

"My child may seem overweight according to the growth charts, but our entire family is big-boned, so I don't think he has a weight problem at all." Pediatricians often hear parents say, "We're not worried about our child's weight. Everyone in our family is big, and we've always been like this." In truth, you need to keep your focus on the growth and body mass index charts. If your child's weight exceeds the normal range for his age and height, he meets the definition of having obesity (see growth charts in Chapter 8). Knowing this, you and your child's pediatrician can address his health risks and help him get back on track to a healthy weight.

There are certain metabolic or hormonal (endocrine) imbalances that often get blamed for weight problems. However, they are responsible for fewer than 1% of the cases of childhood obesity. Yes, hypothyroidism (a deficit in thyroid secretion) and other rarer and more severe genetic and metabolic disorders (eg, Prader-Willi syndrome, Turner syndrome, Cushing syndrome) can cause weight gain (and, in some cases, other severe problems, such as hearing and vision impairments). *You should certainly speak with your child's pediatrician about these concerns and have a complete medical evaluation performed.* But because these syndromes are uncommon, they account for very few cases of obesity. More likely, your child's excess weight is associated with unhealthy eating and activity habits, which we will be addressing in the following chapters of this book.

"Because my child is heavy, he actually needs to eat more food to stay healthy." Based on this belief, many families may give bigger portions to the heavier children because of their size. Nothing could be more counterproductive. You need to rely on the growth charts and your pediatrician's advice and make sure that your child is consuming portion sizes that allow him to maintain an average healthy weight. The sensible nutritional principles described in Chapter 2 should help keep your child's weight just where it should be.

Assessing Your Child's Weight

Beginning with Chapter 2, we'll address your child's weight problem with specific strategies and approaches. We'll start with a discussion of good nutrition and how you can ensure that he eats well-balanced meals that can contribute to normal weight. You'll find some specific recommendations on issues like meal planning, food groups, and portion sizes that can help keep your child traveling along the right path to good health.

Resources

Barlow SE. Expert Committee recommendations regarding the prevention, assessment, and treatment of child and adolescent overweight and obesity: summary report. *Pediatrics.* 2007;120(suppl 4):S164–S192

Copeland KC, Silverstein J, Moore KR, et al. Management of newly diagnosed type 2 diabetes mellitus (T2DM) in children and adolescents. *Pediatrics.* 2013;131(2):364–382

Daniels SR, Hassink SG; American Academy of Pediatrics Committee on Nutrition. The role of the pediatrician in primary prevention of obesity. *Pediatrics.* 2015;136(1):e275–e292

Danielsen YS, Stormark KM, Nordhus IH, et al. Factors associated with low self-esteem in children with overweight. *Obes Facts.* 2012;5(5):722–733

Eisenberg ME, Neumark-Sztainer D, Haines J, Wall M. Weight-teasing and emotional well-being in adolescents: longitudinal findings from Project EAT. *J Adolesc Health.* 2006;38(6):675–683

Fink SK, Racine EF, Mueffelmann RE, Dean MN, Herman-Smith R. Family meals and diet quality among children and adolescents in North Carolina. *J Nutr Educ Behav.* 2014;46(5):418–422

Freedman DS, Dietz WH, Srinivasan SR, Berenson GS. The relation of overweight to cardiovascular risk factors among children and adolescents: the Bogalusa Heart Study. *Pediatrics.* 1999;103(6):1175–1182

Gortmaker SL, Must A, Perrin JM, Sobol AM, Dietz WH. Social and economic consequences of overweight in adolescence and young adulthood. *N Engl J Med.* 1993;329(14):1008–1012

Gortmaker SL, Must A, Sobol AM, Peterson K, Colditz GA, Dietz WH. Television viewing as a cause of increasing obesity among children in the United States, 1986-1990. *Arch Pediatr Adolesc Med.* 1996;150(4):356–362

Halfon N, Larson K, Slusser W. Associations between obesity and comorbid mental health, developmental, and physical health conditions in a nationally representative sample of US children aged 10 to 17. *Acad Pediatr.* 2013;13(1):6–13

Harrison S, Rowlinson M, Hill AJ. "No fat friend of mine": young children's responses to overweight and disability. *Body Image.* 2016;18:65–73

Jaiswal M, Divers J, Dabelea D, et al. Prevalence of and risk factors for diabetic peripheral neuropathy in youth with type 1 and type 2 diabetes: SEARCH for Diabetes in Youth study. *Diabetes Care.* 2017:dc170179

Ogden CL, Carroll MD, Fryar CD, Flegal KM. Prevalence of obesity among adults and youth: United States, 2011–2014. *NCHS Data Brief.* 2015;(219):1–8

Pont SJ, Puhl R, Cook SR, Slusser W; American Academy of Pediatrics Section on Obesity, The Obesity Society. Stigma experienced by children and adolescents with obesity. *Pediatrics.* 2017;140(6):e20173034

Puhl R, Brownell KD. Bias, discrimination, and obesity. *Obes Res.* 2001;9(12):788–805

Rankin J, Matthews L, Cobley S, et al. Psychological consequences of childhood obesity: psychiatric comorbidity and prevention. *Adolesc Health Med Ther.* 2016;7:125–146

Schwimmer JB, Burwinkle TM, Varni JW. Health-related quality of life of severely obese children and adolescents. *JAMA.* 2003;289(14):1813–1819

Serdula MK, Ivery D, Coates RJ, Freedman DS, Williamson DF, Byers T. Do obese children become obese adults? A review of the literature. *Prev Med.* 1993;22(2):167–177

Vila G, Zipper E, Dabbas M, et al. Mental disorders in obese children and adolescents. *Psychosom Med.* 2004;66(3):387–394

Whitaker RC, Wright JA, Pepe MS, Seidel KD, Dietz WH. Predicting obesity in young adulthood from childhood and parental obesity. *N Engl J Med.* 1997;337(13):869–873

Williams J, Wake M, Hesketh K, Maher E, Waters E. Health-related quality of life of overweight and obese children. *JAMA.* 2005;293(1):70–76

Chapter 2
What's to Eat? The Importance of Good Nutrition

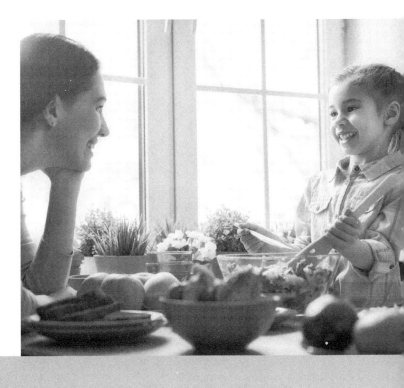

When parents think of the most important strategy for managing their children's weight, their attention often turns to the food they put on their children's plate and perhaps a formal diet or two that they've read about. This book takes a different approach than you might expect. Yes, your child's food consumption is a key factor in attaining a healthy weight. As you'll read, however, we are much more interested in good nutrition than in calorie counting or food restrictions.

The specific nutritional choices you and your child make are crucial, no matter what she weighs. Good nutrition is essential to good health, and the American Academy of Pediatrics (AAP) encourages parents to think of their nutrition decisions as *health* decisions. The nutrition choices for your child today will help determine her health not only now but for the future. If you make an effort to provide primarily healthy meals, beverages, and snacks, you have a much better chance of helping her attain a healthy weight. Remember, your child's pediatrician will help you determine what a healthy weight is for your child, taking into account her age and height.

In this chapter, you will learn healthy eating habits that can last a lifetime. That means staying away from fad diets, including those in which deprivation is front and center. *Never* put your child's health at risk in exchange for weight loss. By familiarizing yourself with ways to optimize her nutrition and creating a health-promoting eating plan for your entire family, you can ensure that your child isn't eating too much or consuming too many calories and is eating the right kinds of foods and beverages in healthy amounts to help her grow. You will read about creating healthy feeding patterns, making smart food-buying decisions, reading and understanding the Nutrition Facts label, and supporting your child's growth.

Supporting Your Child's Growth

As you'll read in this chapter, all children need a variety of foods high in nutritional value—from fruits and vegetables to whole grains, meat or fish, and low-fat dairy—and a sufficient number of calories to grow properly. Infants and adolescents experience the most dramatic surges of childhood growth, but from the moment of birth, *all* children are always growing. In middle childhood, for example, there is a normal weight gain, averaging a little more than 6 pounds a year, that is accompanied by an annual increase in height of slightly more than 2 inches in boys and girls. Later, as puberty approaches, many children experience normal weight gains of 9 to 10 pounds annually. During these kinds of growth spurts, children require more total calories and nutrients. For this reason, even if your child's pediatrician has indicated that weight loss is an appropriate goal, you should *never* place your child on a calorie-restricted diet unless your pediatrician supervises it because strict caloric constraints can keep your child from consuming essential nutrients that she needs to grow. Keep in mind that calories are just a measurement of the energy delivered by food, and she requires energy to fuel her growth and power her physical activity.

At the same time, however, in the midst of the obesity epidemic that you read about in the Introduction, your pediatrician will encourage you to work toward an energy balance in your child's life—that is, balancing her daily calorie consumption with the amount of energy she expends. Food supplies essential nutrients and energy for growth. Food also supplies energy for daily activities and the energy needed to keep the body running. Too little energy and you can compromise growth and activity; too much energy and your body stores it as fat. In past times, this worked out well. Extra energy stored in fat provided energy for when there was famine or not enough to eat. Today, the situation is radically different. Instead of fewer calories, people are eating too many calories on a daily basis and the body keeps storing fat that may never be used. Balancing energy intake and output is something we have to think seriously about. Parents can do this by making sure they are

- Offering food portions that are appropriate for the age of their child (See sample menus in chapters 8–10.)
- Making sure that half the meal is composed of fruits and vegetables (See ChooseMyPlate.gov [**https://www.choosemyplate.gov**].)
- Choosing snacks that are healthy and not high-calorie mini-meals
- Limiting or completely avoiding sugary drinks that add energy without adding nutrients (which can easily upset the healthy energy balance)
- Scheduling meals and snacks instead of allowing grazing
- Turning the television (TV) off during meals to limit unconscious eating

---

WHERE THE AMERICAN ACADEMY OF PEDIATRICS STANDS

The American Academy of Pediatrics feels strongly that healthy eating habits should begin in infancy and continue throughout childhood, adolescence, and beyond. As a parent, you have an enormous influence on your child's eating behaviors that can last a lifetime and can prevent or reduce the risk of obesity. Without your attention focused on what (and how much) she's eating, your child can begin to move in the direction of obesity during her first year of age.

If you are trying to help your child lose weight, *it is very important to do so under the supervision of your child's pediatrician.* Your pediatrician can monitor your child's progress and help ensure that she is maintaining energy balance in a healthy and safe manner. Your pediatrician can help guide you toward feeding your child a balanced diet that, along with regular physical activity, can produce a steady reduction in weight of about 1 pound a week.

Organizing the Nutritional Environment

If you just look around at the food environment, there are high-calorie, salty, and sugary processed foods everywhere—in the grocery store, at the movie theater, at sporting events, in schools, and even at home. You may realize as a parent that you need to take a proactive approach to your family's nutritional environment. Just like you made an effort to childproof your home (putting knifes and other sharp utensils in a latched drawer, keeping matches out of reach and out of sight) when your child was a toddler, you need to create a healthy food environment in which the burden isn't on your child to filter out the bad choices from the good ones. Too many parents have let a nutritional environment at home increasingly fill up with high-calorie snacks in the cupboards and lots of sugar-rich beverages in the refrigerator. They depend on their children to make the most appropriate choices from the array of tempting foods accessible to them.

Figure 2-1 can help you get started on your journey to a healthier pantry and healthier eating. First, make a list and check off which foods are in which columns. Then try to shift your pantry to have more Go foods, with Slow and Whoa as sometimes and infrequent foods.

Figure 2-1. Go, Slow, Whoa Foods

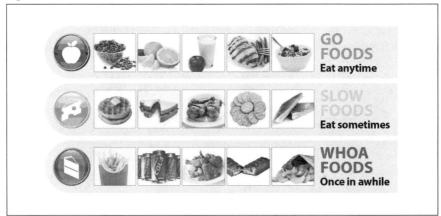

Source: LiveWell Colorado

Go Foods

Go foods are the lowest in fat and sugar, low in calories, and great to eat anytime.

What About Low-fat Milk?

According to the AAP, once your baby is older than 1 year, you may give her whole cow's milk, provided she has a balanced diet of solid foods (cereals, vegetables, fruits, and meats). But limit her intake of milk to 1 quart (32 ounces or 946 mL) per day. More than this can provide too many calories and may decrease her appetite for the other foods she needs.

- Children need a higher fat content in their diet, which is why whole vitamin D milk is recommended for most after 1 year of age.
- If your child is overweight or at risk for being overweight, or if there is a family history of obesity, high blood pressure, or heart disease, your pediatrician may recommend 2% (reduced-fat) milk instead.
- Do not give your baby 1% (low-fat) or nonfat (skim) milk before her second birthday. In addition to needing a higher fat content to maintain normal weight gain, it is also important to help her body absorb vitamins A and D. Also, nonfat milk provides too high a concentration of protein and minerals and should not be given to infants or toddlers younger than 2 years.
- After 2 years of age, you should discuss your child's nutritional needs, including choice of low-fat or nonfat milk products, with your child's pediatrician.
- New research is happening all the time. Right now, there are studies that show whole milk and dairy could move to the Go or Slow column. Check with your pediatrician.

Slow Foods

Slow foods are higher in fat, added sugar, and calories. These should only be eaten sometimes, or less often than Go foods. For parents worried about overweight or obesity in their children, juice should be in the Whoa column.

The AAP recommends that

- Juice should not be introduced to infants before 1 year of age unless clinically indicated.
- Daily intake of juice should be limited to 4 ounces in toddlers aged 1 to 3 years or 4 to 6 ounces for children 4 to 6 years old.
- For 7- to 18-year-olds, juice intake should be limited to 8 ounces or 1 cup of the recommended 2 to 2½ cups of fruit servings per day.
- Toddlers should not be given juice from bottles or easily transportable covered cups that make it easy to consume throughout the day; nor should they be given juice at bedtime.

Whoa Foods

Whoa foods are ones that are highest in fat and added sugar and high in calories. These should only be eaten once in a while and in small portions. Fast food and processed foods fall into this category. Limiting eating out can really help shift your family's diet toward the Go column.

Adopting a structured approach to your child's eating is one way to make sure your child is eating in a healthy way. That means doing some planning for the food that she eats—breakfast, lunch, dinner, and snacks. It may mean using ChooseMyPlate.gov (**https://www.choosemyplate.gov**) and information in this chapter to thoughtfully prepare meals that are balanced and have portion sizes that are appropriate for your child's age. Remember, as her parent, you're in charge of the food environment at home. You should decide which foods come into your home and what will be served and when. When you prepare age-appropriate portions of a nutritionally balanced diet for your child at mealtime and snack time, she can learn to listen to her own hunger signals and choose how much to eat, and you will know that she has the appropriate balance and amount of food needed for her growth and development.

This is an opportunity to set a good example, such as

- Providing at least one fruit or vegetable with every meal
- Putting cut-up fruits and vegetables in the refrigerator for snacks

- Cooking only one helping of food per person, and then serving salad if the family wants extra helpings
- Using smaller dinner plates that are better sized for healthy portions
- Serving one meal for the whole family without cooking special meals for every person
- Scheduling meals and snacks at regular times each day
- Planning meals with a protein (meat, fish, chicken), vegetable, fruit, and dairy serving
- Involving an older child in discussing what she would choose for healthy meals and snacks

Encouraging your children and praising them for making healthy food choices is a good way to help them make this transition.

Meal Planning and ChooseMyPlate.gov

It's important to include a variety of foods in your child's meals to provide essential nutrients and energy that can support normal growth, good health, and sensible weight management.

CHOICES FROM THE MAJOR FOOD GROUPS

Here are examples of foods from the 5 major food groups.

Grains: whole-grain breads, oatmeal, brown rice, pasta, potatoes

Dairy products: milk, yogurt, cheese, cottage cheese

Vegetables: beets, broccoli, carrots, green beans, peas, spinach

Fruits: bananas, apples, pears, strawberries, cantaloupes, watermelons

Meat/protein: lean cuts of beef, skinless poultry, fish, eggs, peanut butter, beans, reduced-fat deli meats, tofu

Nutrition Guidelines

The *2015–2020 Dietary Guidelines for Americans,* 8th Edition, were released by the US departments of Agriculture (USDA) and Health and Human Services to provide scientific information about healthy nutrition to serve as the basis for developing nutrition education materials for the public. Their focus is to help Americans achieve healthier diets to reduce obesity and prevent chronic diseases, such as type 2 diabetes, heart disease, and high blood pressure. The guidelines emphasize the development of a healthy eating pattern, which includes a variety of nutritious foods, like vegetables, fruits, grains, low-fat and fat-free dairy, lean meats and other protein foods, and oils, while limiting saturated fats, trans fats, added sugars, and sodium. A healthy eating pattern can be adapted to a person's taste preferences, traditions, culture, and budget and includes the following foods:

- **Vegetables.** Choose a variety from dark green, red, yellow, and orange.
- **Fruits.** Choose whole fruits when possible.
- **Grains.** Make half of them whole grains.
- **Dairy.** Choose fat-free or low-fat and/or fortified soy beverages.
- **Protein.** Choose from a variety of sources (seafood, lean meats, eggs, beans, nuts, seeds, and soy products).
- **Oils.** Canola, corn, olive, peanut, safflower, soybean, and sunflower oils should replace solid fats.

Creating a Healthy Food Pattern

One way to help ensure that your child has a healthy food pattern is to refer to ChooseMyPlate.gov (**https://www.choosemyplate.gov**) as you're planning and preparing meals and snacks. Created by the USDA, ChooseMyPlate.gov is based on the *Dietary Guidelines for Americans* and focuses on building a healthier eating style for all ages. Some of the basic principles that help families do this are

All food choices matter; focus on the variety and amount of and nutrition in what you eat.

 Choose an eating style that is low in saturated fat, sodium, and added sugars.

3. Make small changes on your way to creating a healthier eating style, such as
   - Try one new vegetable per week.
   - Cut down on sugary beverages and substitute water or milk until your family's beverages are sugar free.
   - Increase the times your family eats a meal together by one time per week until you are eating family meals as a routine.
   - Trade one snack food each shopping trip for more fruits and vegetables.

4. Help each other by supporting healthier eating styles for everyone.
   - Eat one meal together as a family every day.
   - Commit as a family to trying healthier foods.
   - Bring healthier snacks to family gatherings.
   - Split meals to control portions when eating at a restaurant.
   - Decide as a family what food comes into the house. Don't sabotage each other by bringing in sugary drinks, sweets, and high-calorie snacks. ChooseMyPlate.gov (**https://www.choosemyplate.gov**) includes videos of real families making healthy eating a reality, family friendly recipe ideas, information about local foods, and healthy eating on a budget. Table 2-1 provides best choices of foods from each food group and where they are generally located in the grocery store.

Table 2-1. Picky Eater Project Shopping Guide

Food Group	Typical Store Locations	Best Choices
Vegetables and fruits	• Produce aisle • Canned goods • Freezer aisle • Salad bar	Variety! Fresh, frozen, canned, and dried fruits and vegetables. All forms have nearly identical nutrient value. Choose canned fruit in its own juice to minimize added sugars. Choose low-sodium canned vegetables and rinse them first to further decrease sodium content. Watch portion sizes on dried fruit, as they are not only nutrient dense but also high in calories. Whenever possible, it is best to choose locally grown, in-season produce. When deciding whether to buy organic, we suggest using the Environmental Working Group guide at **www.ewg.org.** The "dirty dozen"; in other words, try to buy organic versions of the following foods, because of the relatively high pesticide exposure when grown conventionally: Celery — Sweet bell peppers Peaches — Spinach Strawberries — Tomatoes Apples — Cherries Cherry tomatoes — Cucumbers Nectarines — Grapes (imported) The "clean 15"; the following foods are lowest in pesticides, so you don't need to buy organic: Onions — Sweet peas (frozen) — Cantaloupe (domestic) Avocado — Asparagus — Watermelon Sweet corn (frozen) — Kiwi fruit — Grapefruit Pineapples — Cabbage — Sweet potatoes Mango — Eggplant — Honeydew melon
Grains	• Bakery • Bread aisle • Pasta and rice aisles • Cereal aisle	Try whole-grain bread, brown rice, barley, bulgur, and quinoa. True whole grains will typically have the words *whole grain* as the first ingredient on the package's ingredient list.

Table 2-1 (continued)		
Food Group	**Typical Store Locations**	**Best Choices**
Yogurt and cheese (calcium-rich foods)	• Dairy case • Refrigerated aisle	Prefer nondairy sources of calcium? Try salmon, almonds, Brazil nuts, sunflower seeds, dried beans, or calcium-fortified foods, such as soy milk, tofu, and various breads.
Meat and beans, fish, poultry, eggs, soy, and nuts (protein foods)	• Deli • Meat and poultry case • Seafood counter • Egg case • Canned goods • Salad bar	The leanest forms of red meat are the round and loin cuts. Poultry such as chicken and turkey is an excellent protein source with low-fat content. Include fish in your family's meal plan for optimal health. Fatty fish provide high levels of omega-3 fatty acids, which help boost heart and brain health. These fish include salmon, albacore tuna, and lake trout. Wondering whether it's better to choose farmed or wild-caught fish? The answer of what's best varies. Look up the fish you are considering and get recommendations on what is healthiest and most environmentally conscious at **www.seafoodwatch.org.**

Adapted from Muth ND, Sampson S. *The Picky Eater Project: 6 Weeks to Happier, Healthier Family Mealtimes.* Elk Grove Village, IL: American Academy of Pediatrics; 2017:118–119.

Portion and Serving Sizes

We live in a culture in which many restaurants are renowned for super-sizing virtually every item on their menu and parents often overestimate the amount of food that their children need. That kind of thinking can put children on the fast track to obesity.

Keep in mind that your child does not require the same serving size as an adult. For example, it makes sense that portion sizes should be different for a 5-year-old and a 15-year-old. Even so, many parents are confused over how big their children's servings should be. The key here is to feed age-appropriate portions to your child. As a general guideline, Table 2-2 suggests age-appropriate portions across the various food groups. This is a good way to notice the differences between feeding a toddler and an adolescent. (See also Preventing Choking box in Chapter 9).

Table 2-2. Feeding Guide for Children

Food	2 to 3 (1,000–1,400 kcal)		4 to 6 (1,200–1,800 kcal)		7 to 12 (1,400–2,000 kcal)		Comments
	Portion Size	Daily Amounts	Portion Size	Daily Amounts	Portion Size	Daily Amounts	
Low-fat milk and dairy	½ cup (4 oz)	2½ cups	½–¾ cups (4–6 oz)	2½–3 cups	½–1 cups (4–8 oz)	2½–3 cups	The following may be substituted for ½-cup fluid milk: ½-oz natural cheese, 1-oz processed cheese, ½-cup low-fat yogurt, 2½-tbsp nonfat dry milk.
Meat, fish, poultry, or equivalent	1–2 oz (2–3 tbsp)	2–4 oz	1–2 oz (4–6 tbsp)	3–5 oz	2 oz	4–5½ oz	The following may be substituted for 1-oz meat, fish, or poultry: 1 egg, 1 tbsp peanut butter, ¼-cup cooked beans or peas.
Vegetables (cooked, raw)[a]	2–3 tbsp (few pieces)	1½ cups	4–6 tbsp (few pieces)	1½–2½ cups	¼–½ cup (several pieces)	1½–2½ cups	Include dark-green (1 cup per week) and orange vegetables (3 cups per week) for vitamin A, such as carrots, spinach, broccoli, winter squash, or greens. Limit starch vegetables (potatoes) to 3½ cups weekly.
Fruit (raw[a], canned, juice)	½–1 small 2–3 tbsp 3–4 oz	No more than 4 oz of juice/d	½–1 small 4–6 tbsp 4 oz	No more than 6 oz of juice/d	1 medium ¼–½ cup 4 oz	No more than 8 oz of juice/d	Include one vitamin C-rich fruit, vegetable, or juice, such as citrus juices, orange, grapefruit, strawberries, melon, tomato, or broccoli.

Table 2-2 *(continued)*

Food	Age, y					
	2 to 3 (1,000–1,400 kcal)		4 to 6 (1,200–1,800 kcal)		7 to 12 (1,400–2,000 kcal)	
	Portion Size	Daily Amounts	Portion Size	Daily Amounts	Portion Size	Daily Amounts	Comments
Grain products	½–1 slice	3–5 oz	1 slice	4–6 oz	1 slice	5–6 oz	The following may be substituted for 1 slice of bread: ½-cup spaghetti; macaroni, noodles, or rice; 5 saltines; ½ English muffin or bagel; 1 tortilla; corn grits or posole. Make half of grain intake whole grains.
Whole grain or enriched bread	¼–½ cup	1½–2-oz whole grain	½ cup		½–1 cup		
	½–1 cup		1 cup		1 cup		
Cooked cereal							
Dry cereal							
Oils		4 tsp		4–5 tsp		4–6 tsp	Choose soft margarines. Avoid trans fats. Use liquid vegetable oils rather than solid fats.

Adapted from ChooseMyPlate.gov (http://www.choosemyplate.gov) and the *2010 Dietary Guidelines for Americans*. From American Academy of Pediatrics Committee on Nutrition. *Pediatric Nutrition.* Kleinman RE, Greer FR, eds. 7th ed. Elk Grove Village, IL: American Academy of Pediatrics; 2014:153.
[a] Do not give to young children until they can chew well.

Remember, your child will have her own unique growth pattern, activity, and nutritional needs. For more specifics, ask your child's pediatrician. In fact, you should not make any drastic changes in the amount your child eats until you discuss it with your pediatrician.

One way to help avoid serving excessively large portion sizes to your child is to make sure that there are a variety of food groups on her plate. If you serve her a protein source, such as chicken; 2 vegetables; and pasta for dinner, there simply won't be room on her plate to overdo it on the pasta, for example. Your job as a parent is to provide healthy portions for your child's age, and your child's job is to eat to satisfy her hunger. Telling her to clean her plate or eat her vegetables so she can have dessert defeats the purpose of putting her in charge of her own hunger cues.

Some children race through their meals and have no idea how much they're eating. By slowing down the pace, a child will be able to judge whether she is still hungry. She'll be giving her brain the chance to recognize that she has eaten enough to feel satisfied, and when she's no longer hungry, she's more likely to stop eating. Also, by taking smaller bites and chewing her food thoroughly, she'll enjoy her food more. Talking helps to slow down the eating process and also allows people to find out what is going on in each other's lives and enjoy one another's company. The best way to help your child slow down is to be a good role model yourself.

By eating together as a family, you can help your child with healthy eating habits as well as provide valuable family together time. Keep meals pleasant and focus on the positives. *Remember that your job is to provide nutritional, well-balanced meals in the proper portions, and your child will decide what to eat.* Overfocusing on food and eating can be replaced by finding out what happened at school and with their friends and leave time for family interactions.

NUTRITIONAL BALANCE

Nutritional balance is the key. All healthy foods contain essential nutrients for your child's growth and health. The key to a healthy weight is choosing the appropriate amounts of each food. Focusing on only one food as the culprit can lead to an imbalance in meeting nutritional needs. That's not to say that you don't have to watch out for excess snack foods, sugared beverages, and large portions, but try to offer a balanced approach and limit high-calorie sweets and snacks by only having these foods in small amounts for special occasions. Rely more often on foods like

- Fresh fruits and vegetables
- Whole-grain breads and cereals
- Low-fat and nonfat dairy products (eg, milk, yogurt)
- Moderate portions of skim-milk cheeses
- Lean meats (eg, chicken, turkey, lean beef cuts, lean pork cuts)
- Fish

Here are some healthier options when it comes to desserts/snacks.

- Pretzels, baked tortilla chips, and baked potato chips
- Frozen fruit bars and angel food cake instead of rich, creamy desserts

Making Smart Shopping Choices

If you're like most parents, you probably don't have time to do as much menu planning as you'd like. You may feel that the decisions you make in the supermarket occur in the spur of the moment much too often. Most supermarkets carry thousands of food items on their shelves, and impulse buying can be risky. You may end up purchasing foods that you had no intention of buying.

For that reason, it pays to have a plan. Find a few minutes before you shop to make a list of the basic items you need, concentrating on the healthy foods described in this chapter. It's also a good idea to shop at a market that you're familiar with, where you know the location of most of the foods you want. You'll spend less time browsing down the aisles, where you may find and choose foods that your family doesn't need.

When you enter the market, concentrate first on shopping along its outer borders, where most stores keep fresh fruits and vegetables, dairy products, and meats. Packaged items, which are often higher in calories, tend to be on interior shelves of the store. Invite your older child to shop with you to learn about nutrition labels and be an active participant in selecting healthy foods. Just prior to purchasing your groceries, spend a moment that might be called "Checking Out Before Checkout"; look into your cart, make sure that what is in your cart are the healthy items you actually want, and put back the rest.

Healthy food selection is only the first step in this process. Once you're in the kitchen and preparing meals, be sure to trim all visible fat from meat and remove the skin from chicken before cooking. Also, use cooking techniques such as broiling, roasting, and steaming that call for little or no fat. If your family likes butter or margarine on cooked vegetables, try to add only small amounts or use healthy oils, such as a bit of olive oil or pesto sauce. Including younger children and adolescents in cooking tasks appropriate to their age is a great way to get them interested in new and healthy foods you want to try as a family and gives them a lifelong health-building skill.

The Nutrition Facts Label

The following exercise may be helpful to you to test your label-reading skills and give you a glimpse into your own health literacy. Review the sample Nutrition Facts label for a pint of ice cream in Figure 2-2, and then answer the questions that follow. The answers and scoring key are listed on page 34.

Nutrition Label Questions

 If you eat the entire container how many calories will you eat?

If you are allowed to eat 60 g of carbohydrates as a snack, how much ice cream could you have? (Answer in a measure other than serving size.)

**Figure 2-2. Sample Nutrition Facts Label
for 1 Pint of Ice Cream**

Nutrition Facts

Serving Size	1/2 cup
Servings per container	4

Amount per serving

Calories 250	Fat Cal 120

	%DV
Total Fat 13g	20%
Sat Fat 9g	40%
Cholesterol 28mg	12%
Sodium 55mg	2%
Total Carbohydrate 30g	12%
Dietary Fiber 2g	
Sugars 23g	
Protein 4g	8%

* Percent Daily Values (DV) are based on a 2,000 calorie diet. Your daily values may be higher or lower depending on your calorie needs.

Ingredients: Cream, Skim Milk, Liquid Sugar, Water, Egg Yolks, Brown Sugar, Milkfat, Peanut Oil, Sugar, Butter, Salt, Carrageenan, Vanilla Extract.

Adapted or reprinted with permission from Quick Assessment of Literacy in Primary Care: The Newest Vital Sign, 3.6, 2005, Vol 3, No 6, *Annals of Family Medicine.* Copyright © 2005 American Academy of Family Physicians. All Rights Reserved.

 Your doctor advises you to reduce the amount of saturated fat in your diet. You usually have 42 g of saturated fat each day, which includes 1 serving of ice cream. If you stop eating ice cream, how many grams of saturated fat would you be consuming each day?

 If you usually eat 2,500 calories in a day, what percentage of your daily value of calories will you be eating if you eat 1 serving?

 Pretend that you are allergic to the following substances: penicillin, peanuts, latex gloves, and beestings. Is it safe for you to eat this ice cream?

6 If you answered no to question 5, why not?

Answer Key

1 1,000 calories

2 The following responses are correct:
- 1 cup
- Any amount up to 1 cup
- Half the container

3 33 g

4 10%

5 No

6 Because it has peanut oil

Scoring

If you got 4 or more answers correct, congratulations! You are on your way to being a champion label reader. For more detailed information, see the US Food and Drug Administration article "How to Understand and Use the Nutrition Facts Label" at **https://www.fda. gov/food/ingredientspackaginglabeling/labelingnutrition/ucm274593.htm.**

Eating on the Run

You know the feeling—you're rushing in the morning to get your children off to school, you're hurrying in the afternoon to drive them to soccer practice, and you're racing home from work in the evening to make sure they have time for a study session at a friend's house.

When something's got to give in a tight schedule, it's often family meals. Many families never sit down to eat together even once during the day. When everyone is eating on the run or the kids are having some of their meals or snacks away from home (eg, at an early child care and education center, at friends' homes), that's when healthy foods can give way to the easier, higher fat, higher calorie choices. Sound familiar?

Even if there never seem to be enough hours in the day for your family to eat as healthfully as you'd like, don't despair. Here are some suggestions to help keep your child and your family on the right track.

- Plan ahead for those times when you know you're going to be busy. It may mean spending time on the weekend preparing meals for the upcoming weekdays, but it will be worth it!
- Sit together at the table for meals as a family whenever possible to eat and talk together.
- Discuss how the family can decrease eating out at fast-food restaurants—maybe by simplifying meals or cooking together to lighten the work.
- Fix breakfast the night before. You can precook hard-boiled eggs or have your child's favorite cold cereal already in the bowl and the fresh fruit sliced and ready to go at the crack of dawn.
- Keep things simple. You don't have to cook an elaborate dinner every night. For example, why not prepare a bowl of soup, a sandwich, and a salad, topping the meal off with a piece of fruit and a glass of milk, on evenings when you're particularly rushed? It will provide your child with a nutritious meal without pushing yourself to the point of collapse. The key is to make good nutritional choices, no matter how simple or extravagant the meal is.
- When your child spends time at friends' homes, call the parents of your child's friends and offer to send over healthy foods or snacks for all the kids. Turkey sandwiches or apples may keep your child from grabbing higher fat choices that her friends might otherwise offer.
- For a child who goes to an early child care and education center, family child care, or after-school program or eats at the school cafeteria, find out what the nutritional environment is like, including food and beverages. If the menu relies too often on cheeseburgers and French fries, your child needs to bring her own meals and snacks from home. At the same time, talk to your school or child care administrator about improving the nutritional choices. Don't forget about the school

vending machines, either; if they're weighed down with candy and soft drinks, you and other parents should lobby for an improvement in the available selections.

The Perils of Fast Food

Fast-food restaurants have permeated every corner of the United States and are probably in the consciousness of nearly every US child. Many TV advertisements for these eating establishments are targeted specifically at children, and so are the promotional toys and the playgrounds that are part of the restaurant offerings. As a result, millions of kids persuade their parents to line up their cars at the drive-through window several days a week—and in a fast-paced world in which adults and children alike often seem to have too much squeezed into their days, parents are only too happy to give in to the convenience of the local fast-food restaurant from time to time. In fact, according to the USDA, in 2014 Americans spent approximately 50% of their total food expenditures on food away from home, surpassing at-home food sales for the first time. According to a 2013 Gallup poll, 8 in 10 Americans reported eating at fast-food restaurants at least monthly, with almost half saying they eat fast food at least weekly. Only 4% say they never eat at fast-food restaurants. Yes, it's possible to make nutritious fast-food selections. But let's face it—there are many more high-fat, high-sugar, high-calorie choices, from hamburgers to fries to shakes, often served in king-sized portions that can sabotage your child's best efforts to control her weight. Fast foods often don't supply a healthy balance of vitamins and minerals and are frequently very high in salt.

When you do take the kids to a fast-food restaurant, talk with them in advance about making healthier choices. You can reduce the effect of impulsive fast-food choices by planning ahead.

- A grilled or charbroiled chicken sandwich (without the skin and mayonnaise).

- A regular-sized hamburger (not the large one with all the fixings). Lettuce and tomato are good and make it more filling compared with cheese and bacon.
- A salad with a small amount of salad dressing (or ask for it on the side).
- A plain baked potato (perhaps topped with vegetables from the salad bar).
- Nonfat (skim) or 1% (low-fat) milk rather than a sugary, high-calorie, high-fat shake or soda.
- If your child must have fries, divide a single order among several members of the family. (Some chains now cook their French fries in vegetable oil rather than animal fat.)
- Use the nutritional content charts that are available in the restaurant (you may have to ask for one) to help make healthier choices.

Your child may love fast-food fare, and it can seem like the breather you need at the end of an exhausting day. But if you do the math, you might be surprised that fast-food dining is expensive. If it costs $20 or $25 to feed a family of 4 at a fast-food restaurant, and if you eat there 3 or 4 times a week, that can take a supersized bite out of the family budget. Ask yourself whether you could take that same money and buy more nutritious food for your family. On those days when the family does eat out, avoid fast food and consider splitting portions, which are often too large. It is wise to steer clear of buffets that can tempt everyone to eat too large of portions and second helpings.

One other important suggestion: Eat as many of your meals at home as possible or pack healthier foods for when you are on the run. When you or another adult in the home does the cooking, there is more control over what your child eats. Turn those trips to the fast-food restaurant into a once-in-a-while experience, not an everyday outing. When you have the opportunity to sit down for a meal as a family, grab it.

The Power of Incremental Changes

A lot of diet programs ask people to transform the way they eat and make these major changes overnight. Not surprisingly, most individuals have trouble sticking to those kinds of dramatic shifts in their diets, particularly over the long term. Eating habits develop over many years, and they can be hard to change.

For that reason, the recommendations in this book are quite different. When it comes to your child, you need to help her make *gradual, small* changes in her eating habits over time. Introduce 1 or 2 changes a week. Consider making one change at a time and do not take on another change until the first one is mastered and going well. She'll find those kinds of changes—a little at a time—are the easiest kinds to make. Involve your child in deciding which change to work on first. This helps her know that you value her input and helps her feel part of the family team.

You've already read some ideas to help make this transition in slow and steady increments. For example, it could mean eating out at restaurants less often—perhaps twice a week rather than 4 or 5 times a week. Or you might order a small hamburger or grilled chicken sandwich for your child rather than the titanic-sized burger. Here are some other suggestions for incremental dietary changes.

- Introduce new, healthier foods over time. Some children are resistant to try any new food; it may take multiple attempts before they develop a taste for it.
- Evaluate what snack foods your family is eating, and gradually move them in the direction of healthier alternatives—for example, unsalted pretzels rather than potato chips, air-popped popcorn instead of cookies, and low-fat yogurt bars (without added sugar) or yogurt with fresh fruit instead of ice cream.

- Serve salads more often, and choose low-fat salad dressing. Teach children about an appropriate amount of salad dressing to use and how they can order it on the side at restaurants.
- When making sandwiches, use low-fat meats (eg, turkey, ham) and see if your child notices the difference.
- Switch from mayonnaise and other high-fat spreads to reduced-fat varieties. Use spreads sparingly and teach your child to do the same.
- Try out a child-friendly vegetarian recipe for spaghetti or lasagna, using vegetables instead of meat, along with lower fat cheeses.
- Swap out sour cream with Greek yogurt.
- Choose egg whites instead of the whole egg.
- Gradually substitute water or milk for sugary drinks.

All in the Family

As we'll emphasize throughout this book, helping your child achieve a healthy weight should be a family project. It's logical that you can't expect your child to change her eating habits on her own while others in the household are showing no self-restraint and continuing to reach for candy and ice cream. Children are just too smart to accept a "Do as I say, not as I do" attitude from their parents and other family members.

To most effectively help your child, your *entire* family needs to get on board. That means modeling healthy eating behaviors that you want your child to adopt, now and in the future. It means recruiting all the adults in your child's life, as well as your other children, as active members of the support team who are setting a good example, day by day. If everyone adopts the same eating plan, your child will feel supported. If family members are doing their own things, you risk making your child struggle with her weight and feel singled out, isolated, and even resentful, and you may increase the chances of failure.

Now, what if you have a child in your family who has obesity, but your other children do not? How do you explain to a child with normal

CHOOSING HEALTHY SNACKS

If the snacks at your home have usually been cookies, doughnuts, and soft drinks, it's time for a change. One or 2 snacks a day are an important part of your child's overall nutrition, so you need to make them just as nutritionally sound as her regular meals, while contributing to an overall program aimed at stabilizing or losing weight. Planning snacks ahead of time is helpful—prepackage some appropriate servings to have ready for kids in their lunches or when they get home from school. This is an opportunity to teach healthy choices and practices.

If you keep the pantry, refrigerator, and kitchen table stocked with plenty of healthy snacks from a variety of foods, that's what she'll reach for. Of course, occasional snacks like ice cream are fine. But wouldn't it be great if your child learned that fruits and vegetables were the first choice for snacks? Think of the nutrition she would be getting.

Here are some suggestions for those snacks that your child typically grabs on her own.

- Fruit
- Low-fat/frozen yogurt
- Celery stalks
- Low-fat oatmeal cookies
- Cucumber slices
- Frozen bananas
- Baked potato chips
- Bran muffins
- Fresh strawberries
- Air-popped popcorn
- Low-fat cheeses
- Frozen juice bars (without added sugar)
- Crackers
- Sugar-free cereals
- Unsalted pretzels
- Homemade granola

Adding a protein food with these snacks can make them more satisfying. Try adding a boiled egg, cheese stick, yogurt, natural peanut butter, or nuts (if your child is old enough that choking is not a concern).

weight that the entire family is adopting a new way of eating, even if she has no need to lose or stabilize weight herself? Here is the approach that we recommend. Explain that the entire family is going to work at getting *healthier* and that the nutritional changes being made are for the well-being of the *entire* family, from the thinnest to the most overweight ("We're going to have strawberries for dessert tonight instead of chocolate cake because it's a lot healthier for *all* of us."). You can also mention that your approach to healthier eating is a way for you all to be aware of smart choices when it comes to maintaining a healthy weight.

At the same time, turn mealtime into family time whenever possible. Try eating most of your meals together. Children learn more about good food choices and healthy nutrition when family members join one another for breakfast, lunch, and dinner. Research also shows that when families eat together, kids eat more vegetables and fruits and consume fewer fried foods and sugary drinks.

As you use the recommendations in this chapter to change the way your whole family eats, you will find that this new nutritional approach becomes easier with time. Remember, you don't need to count calories or fat grams, and you don't need to panic if your child has a bad day or even a bad week in making healthy choices. A little backsliding isn't going to derail a good eating plan if you help her get back on track as soon as possible. Remember that energy balance is the long-term goal.

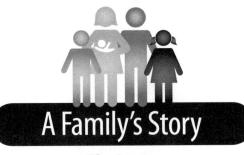

A Family's Story

The Letter

Jean and Bob are busy parents. Jean is a kindergarten teacher and Bob manages the local hardware store. They have 2 children, 10-year-old Jerry and 8-year-old Melissa. They work hard to keep their family healthy, keeping up with well-child visits to the pediatrician, making sure the children brush their teeth, and ensuring they get enough sleep at night. When they received a letter from school that indicated Jerry's body mass index was at the 95th percentile and he was at risk for health problems related to his weight, they were shocked. The letter from the school suggested that they see their pediatrician, so Bob made an appointment immediately.

In the meantime, Jean thought back to some of the family's eating patterns. She remembered when the kids were infants, how careful she and Bob had been about what they ate, providing fresh food and avoiding sugary cereals and drinks. But things had only gotten busier and busier since then: Bob's job had gotten more demanding; Jean began spending more time taking care of her mother, who had developed heart disease; and, of course, nothing was slowing down for Jerry and Melissa. With the appointment for a visit with Jerry's pediatrician on her mind, Jean started to notice that Jerry's portions were as big as his father's and that it had become a routine for the family to eat fast food 1 or 2 nights per week, especially on the days Bob worked late. Jean also noticed that Melissa was into sugary cereal with her favorite cartoon character on the front.

Jean and Bob evaluating their family's food patterns was a great starting point to gather information to eventually share with their pediatrician. This information could help pinpoint some of the causes of Jerry's weight gain and possibly assist the pediatrician in providing solutions to help Jerry manage his weight, as well as provide ways to help Melissa and the rest of the family develop better eating habits.

Key Points to Remember

 Food decisions are health decisions, and every time you plan, shop for, and cook a healthy meal you are contributing to your child's and family's overall health.

 Small changes completed over time add up to big accomplishments; start small and keep going!

❸ Plan for stressful times with precooked dinners in the freezer and simplified meal plans.

❹ Involve the whole family in your quest for healthier eating. Pick out times to eat together, and create special healthy meals the family cooks together.

Resources

American Academy of Pediatrics. Why formula instead of cow's milk? HealthyChildren Web site. https://www.healthychildren.org/English/ages-stages/baby/feeding-nutrition/Pages/Why-Formula-Instead-of-Cows-Milk.aspx. Updated November 21, 2015. Accessed October 30, 2017

Dugan A. Fast food still a major part of US diet. Gallup Web site. http://www.gallup.com/poll/163868/fast-food-major-part-diet.aspx. Published August 6, 2013. Accessed October 30, 2017

Fink SK, Racine EF, Mueffelmann RE, Dean MN, Herman-Smith R. Family meals and diet quality among children and adolescents in North Carolina. *J Nutr Educ Behav.* 2014;46(5):418–422

Heyman MB, Abrams SA; American Academy of Pediatrics Section on Gastroenterology, Hepatology, and Nutrition and Committee on Nutrition. Fruit juice in infants, children, and adolescents: current recommendations. *Pediatrics.* 2017;139(6):e20170967

US Department of Agriculture. Food expenditures. https://www.ers.usda.gov/data-products/food-expenditures.aspx. Updated October 26, 2017. Accessed October 30, 2017

Chapter 3

Physical Activity, Sedentary Behavior, and Sleep

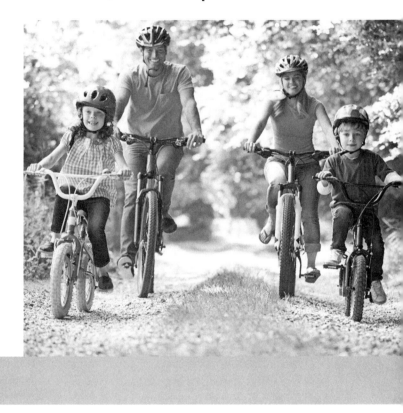

A generation ago, most parents didn't give much thought to whether their children were physically active. In many families, the kids came home from school, had a snack, and then headed outdoors to play with friends until they were called in for dinner. Most children, it seemed, were constantly active without much or any coaxing. When it came to indoor activities, the action didn't stop, as hide-and-go-seek, imaginary play, and indoor tag seemed to come naturally.

Times have changed. Today, millions of US children are driven to school and just about everywhere else they need to go. At school, they may spend more time sitting and less time moving, thanks to cutbacks in physical education (PE) classes. At home, their parents may not give them household chores that could keep them active. And they've traded in afternoons at the playground for hours spent playing video games or watching television (TV). Unfortunately, children are paying the price for all that time spent operating the TV remote and video game controller. As you've already read, there's an epidemic of obesity and an increase in sedentary time, and the waning interest in physical activity is one of the reasons why. After all, with children spending an average of 3 hours a day in front of the TV or computer screen, they're not playing, running, jumping, or otherwise being physically active. Television watching is a completely sedentary activity (or inactivity, to be more accurate). To make matters worse, many children snack while they're sitting in front of the TV. Having a TV in their bedroom, as so many children do, can interfere with needed sleep (a risk factor for obesity). In addition, there's minimal fresh fruit and vegetable advertising on TV, while the marketing of fast food and sugared cereals and drinks is all too common. That's why the American Academy of Pediatrics (AAP) urges you to help your child understand the importance of physical activity and encourage him to choose to be active every day.

Physical Activity = Better Health

Pediatricians continue to be disturbed by the trends they're seeing in the levels of physical activity of children, which appear to be headed in the wrong direction. As you can see in Figure 3-1, only 27% of boys and 22.5% of girls engage in 60 minutes or more of physical activity every day. Particularly with weight management as a goal, those numbers aren't enough to help in maintaining a healthy weight.

Not only will regular physical activity help your child lose weight and maintain that weight loss, but it has many other benefits. For example, if your child exercises regularly, he'll have

- Stronger bones and joints
- Greater muscle strength
- A decrease in body fat
- Improved flexibility
- A healthier cardiovascular system (thus reducing his risk of developing heart disease and high blood pressure)
- A reduced likelihood of developing diabetes
- More energy and less stress
- Improvements in self-confidence and self-esteem
- Greater social acceptance by physically active peers because they have more physical skills
- Opportunities to make new friends through participation in sports and games
- Better concentration at school

Getting Started

It is important to get a clear picture of your child's activity level, sedentary time, and sleep—and whether he needs to change course. Is he watching too much TV? Is he spending too little time playing outdoors after school or on weekends? Is he getting too little sleep? To get the picture you may want to keep track the number of minutes

Figure 3-1. Percentage of Youth Who Were Physically Active, by Number of Days Per Week and Sex: United States, 2012

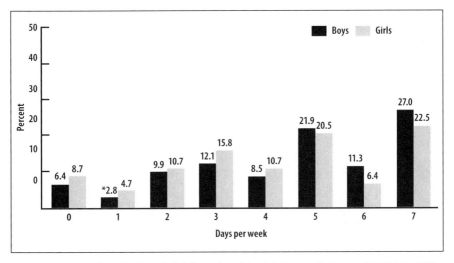

*Does not meet standard of statistical reliability and precision (relative standard error of ≥30% but <40%).
NOTES: Physically active is defined as engaging in any kind of moderate-to-vigorous physical activity, including activities both in school and outside of school, that increased heart rate and made breathing harder some of the time for at least 60 minutes. Weighted percentages are shown. Access data table for Figure 1 at: http://www.cdc.gov/nchs/data/databriefs/db141_table.pdf#1.
SOURCE: CDC/NCHS, National Health and Nutrition Examination Survey and National Youth Fitness Survey, 2012.

spent on physical activity, screen time, free play, homework, and other activities, for 1 week (Table 3-1).

As the parent, you are the major motivator to help your child get moving. Emphasize that he should be engaging in some physical activity every day. In fact, it should become as routine a part of his life as brushing his teeth and sleeping. You can use Table 3-1 to see where improvements can be made.

So where do you begin? How much time does your child need to spend being active and how intense does this activity need to be? The answers to these questions may be different for your child than it is for another boy or girl. If your child has been completely sedentary, with no PE classes at school, no outdoor play, no extracurricular physical activities,

Table 3-1. Sedentary Time and Activity Tracker

	Homework	Screen Time (ie, TV, phone, or computer)	Family Activity (Indicate if active or sedentary.)	Walking	Recess/ Free Play	Physical Education	Outdoor Play	Sports	Indoor Exercise/ Chores	Sleep
Monday										
Tuesday										
Wednesday										
Thursday										
Friday										
Saturday										
Sunday										

and hours of screen time every day, his starting point should be different than that of a fairly active child. There are plenty of activities that he can choose from, and he should begin to slowly and gradually pick up the pace.

Let's say that your child decides to try taking walks or hikes with an older sibling through a nearby park. If he is very out of shape or has trouble imagining doing any walking at all, encourage him to set a goal of walking for only 1 minute at a time ("Can you walk for just 60 seconds?"). Once he realizes that 1 minute is an attainable target, have him increase his walking sessions progressively, to 2 minutes each time, and then 3 minutes, and so on, until he's walking for 30 minutes or more. If your child is already in good shape, he may want to start with a 15-minute walk and then increase it in 5-minute increments to 20 minutes, 25 minutes, and beyond. The ultimate goal is to have him spend 1 hour being active each day.

To most of us, a minute or two of walking doesn't sound like much. In fact, many adolescents and adults think that exercise doesn't count unless it's intense and even hurts (as the cliché goes, "No pain, no gain").

TALKING WITH YOUR CHILD'S PEDIATRICIAN

Before your child moves from a sedentary to a more active way of life, and particularly if he has any health problems, talk with your child's pediatrician. Your pediatrician will be able to tell you how to ensure that exercising is a safe and enjoyable experience for your child. Above all, ask the pediatrician whether your child has any physical limitations or any accommodations that are needed to participate or allow regular activity that you need to keep in mind. For example, many parents think that children who have asthma can't play outdoors on a cold day, or they'll risk having asthmatic episodes. Your pediatrician can help you and your child plan for safe outdoor activity by including this option in your child's asthma plan. Children with special health care needs are often more at risk for obesity and need to be physically active. Check with your pediatrician for community opportunities for activities geared to your child and recommendations for activities to be included in your child's individualized education program (IEP) for school.

But for a child trying to lose weight, every little bit of activity helps, whether it's a short walk to the school bus stop or a climb up a flight of stairs at school. Ultimately, once your child gets into better shape, you can encourage him to increase the duration and intensity of his activity, but the most important thing is that he just gets moving and does it regularly.

What Activity Should Your Child Choose?

There are a lot of avenues for your child to pursue in the quest to become more active. From Little League baseball to ballet lessons, shooting a basketball to bicycling, he has many options to choose from. Community organizations can be great resources for children, including children with special health care needs. And that's the key—*your child,* not you, should be the person making the choice. If he's going to stay active long term, he needs to select something that he likes and will keep doing. Of course, you need to be able to support whatever his choses financially and spend the time it will take to drive him back and forth.

Here are some ideas to get you and your child started. Remember that not all sports or activities will have your child running around for the entire practice or game, but if he is just getting started, any activity that he enjoys can be a great starting place. Check the box next to each activity your child might like to participate in.

☐ Active play (with friends)	☐ Track	☐ Mom/Dad tots play group	☐ Supervised weight lifting
☐ Soccer	☐ Lacrosse	☐ Golf	☐ Yoga classes
☐ Baseball/softball	☐ Frisbee	☐ After-school boys/girls club	☐ Special Olympics
☐ Volleyball	☐ Tennis	☐ Boy/Girl Scouts	☐ Add your own here.
☐ Basketball	☐ Gymnastics	☐ School walking/ running club	_____
☐ Swimming	☐ Dance/hip hop		_____
☐ Archery	☐ Ice-skating		

It's important that parents not micromanage their children's physical activities. Some children enjoy organized activity, while others prefer outdoor free play individually or with a group, for which they're left to their own devices on how they'll be active. Free play can be a powerful form of exercise, contributing to the development of motor skills and serving as a great outlet for your child's energy. As a society, we overlook the value of this kind of active play, even though the AAP recommends *only* free play, rather than team sports, up to the age of 6 years. Whether you live in a city or rural area, find a park, playground, or other outdoor area where your child can safely engage in individual and group play.

For your preschool-aged child, you can make sure that some balls and other play equipment are available whenever your child goes outside, but let him decide exactly what he wants to do. Some play ideas for your preschool child can include

- Playing with supervision on the backyard swing set
- Joining a gymnastics program
- Installing a sandbox and having toys in the backyard
- Playing a game of hide-and-go-seek together
- Planning a visit to the zoo

Parents often find it helpful to give their children 3 or 4 activity options from which to choose or try, or they might ask them what choices they'd like available.

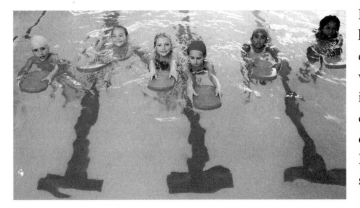

Pose a question like this to your child: "If you weren't watching TV, what could you be doing instead?" Don't be surprised if you initially get a blank stare from him; give him some concrete alternatives: "Could you jump rope? Or play tennis? Or go in-line skating? Or go for a brisk walk?" The most powerful influence on a child is role modeling by a parent. Let your child see you engaging in physical activity, putting down the phone to go outside, or making plans for a parent–child game of catch. It's important to engage your child and let him choose what would be a fun physical activity to do with you. You may be surprised at what he comes up with!

Try saying: "Here are a few activities you could do this afternoon. You could swim, go bowling with your brother, go for a walk with me, or play with your soccer ball in the backyard. Which one would you like to do?"

On the other hand, if you *insist* that your child participate in an activity that he finds boring or grueling—"Jimmy, it's time to walk on the treadmill!"—he'll probably lose interest quickly and end up in front of the TV, or learn to dread the activity if it is forced on him. If you provide him the opportunity to participate in an activity that he enjoys, he's likely to keep doing it.

What about organized sports, like soccer teams and Little League? They're fine for children aged 6 years and older who want to join in, but it's important to have realistic expectations. Your aim should be for your child to be physically active and enjoy the experience, not necessarily excel as the best player on the team. You shouldn't be trying to create an elite athlete, and if he chooses to move from one sport to another rather than concentrating only on one, that's fine. For example, if he shows an interest in a basketball league, great—but if he also wants to learn how to ski when winter comes around, all the better. Let him explore different activities. He'll develop a wide variety of physical skills and, more importantly, he'll keep moving.

Here are some other things to keep in mind when selecting activities with your child.

- Anything that involves movement qualifies as physical activity. It doesn't have to push your child to the point of collapse to contribute to his efforts at weight management.

WHAT'S RIGHT FOR YOUR CHILD?

There's no scarcity of activities that you can make available to your child, and *all* kids can find some form of exercise that they enjoy, even if they tell you that they'd much rather sit and watch TV. You'll find many of these options mentioned throughout this chapter. You can also use your imagination to add to the list of appropriate choices for your own child, perhaps including hiking, working in the school or community garden, snorkeling, gymnastics, stair climbing, or playing with a hula hoop. Consider adopting a family dog if it's within the family budget and pet allergies are not present. Walking the dog as a family can allow for further family communication. Also, when old enough, allow your child to walk the dog as part of his assigned chores. You could also buy him a basketball and put up a hoop in your driveway. Remember, even household chores—from raking leaves to vacuuming the house to washing the car—qualify as physical activity as long as they keep your child moving.

Don't overlook youth activities sponsored by your community's parks and recreation department, which might include volleyball, badminton, or table tennis. Encourage your child to stay active by giving him tools that promote activities, like a catcher's mitt, running shoes, or dance lessons. At his birthday parties, incorporate some physical activity, perhaps by taking his friends and him to play miniature golf or planning a trip to the batting cages to swing at baseballs. Also, keep in mind that there are sports that he can develop a love for and continue doing throughout his lifetime. If you can get your child interested in an activity like this when he's young, exercise and fitness are more likely to become a habit that lasts for many decades. In fact, the American Academy of Pediatrics recommends that physical education programs in schools emphasize lifetime sports (as well as activities that are not just for the best athletes). These include

▹ Swimming	▹ Basketball	▹ In-line and ice-skating
▹ Golf	▹ Bowling	▹ Bicycling
▹ Tennis	▹ Skiing	▹ Track
▹ Walking	▹ Martial arts	

No matter what activity your child chooses, whether it burns lots of body fat or just a little, it is better than just sitting. That's the message to communicate to a child who wants to lose weight, as well as one who would like to maintain a healthy weight.

■ When you present your child with alternatives or options for activities, create the boundaries of acceptable choices. Perhaps joining the hockey team is too expensive for your family budget—not only the sign-up fee but the cost of the skates and other equipment. There are plenty of other choices that can be within your family's financial means.

THE ACTIVITY PYRAMID

To help your child choose physical activities that are right for him, you might try using the Activity Pyramid. It is a visually appealing way to teach children the importance of physical activity, incorporating it into your daily routine, and making it fun.

As you can see, the Activity Pyramid divides activities into 5 groups, each of which represents a particular level or type of movement or exercise. For example

▸ **Base Level:** The greatest amount of space in the pyramid, its base, is devoted to activities that should be done most frequently. These are unstructured, from playing outside to playing with your pet, and should be part of a daily routine.

▸ **Middle Level:** Moving up the pyramid, the next level includes 3 ways to be active. Free play includes activities that are unstructured, like hide-and-seek or flying a kite, that can be done individually or with family and friends. Group play is more structured opportunities to play games with rules, sports, or dance. Family play includes all the activities families can do to enjoy their time together, like walking in the park or tossing a Frisbee.

▸ **Top Level:** Finally, the top level shows activities (or, more specifically, inactivities) that children may become involved in, from TV watching to playing video games; the key is to do these inactivities less often.

Bear in mind that the pyramid is there to give you suggestions for thinking about your child's activities that you all can work on, as well as to provide options he can engage in with friends. When he is just starting to incorporate physical activity into his life, he won't be doing everything on the pyramid. But he can get started by selecting activities he enjoys from various levels of the pyramid.

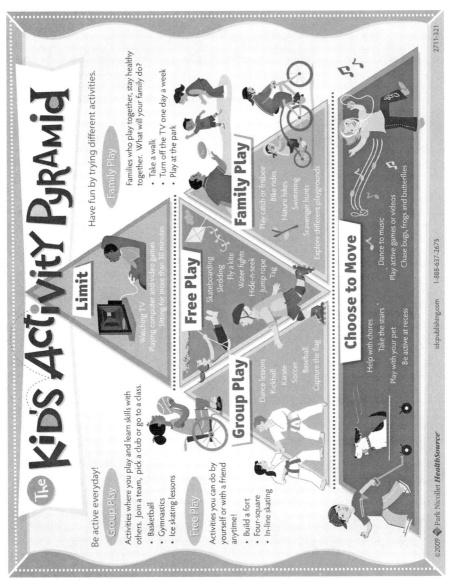

The Kid's Activity Pyramid © 2009 International Diabetes Center, Minneapolis, MN.
Used with permission.

- While many kids love being active with others, some children may feel self-conscious or embarrassed about participating in group sports. They may be more inclined to choose an activity that they can do on their own. Another approach is to plan physical activities for your child together with a special friend or sibling with whom he feels comfortable.
- Above all, the activity must be fun, whether or not your child is successful. Learning new physical skills can be a source of confidence and pride for your child.

Physical Activity and Your Child's Safety

Do you live in a neighborhood where you aren't comfortable having your child play outdoors unsupervised? These days, millions of parents feel this way. They're convinced that it simply isn't safe for their children to be active outdoors, particularly on their own. And if parents are working during the day, it's not surprising that they don't want their kids spending time outside when they're not home.

One of the best options for you to explore is whether there's a formal after-school program in your neighborhood in which your child can participate that involves physical activity. For example, call the YMCA in your community or the Boys & Girls Club. Enroll your child in a dance class to learn jazz or tap. Support your child in joining a youth bowling league. Be on the lookout for activities that are available in your community that include boys and girls. Remember that participation is the key. Your child will be supervised while staying active, and you can pick him up on the way home from work.

If your child is old enough to stay home by himself in the afternoons until you return from work, help him plan that time in advance. He doesn't have to watch TV, play video games, or eat. In fact, there are many ways in which your child can stay active indoors. Sit down with him and let him choose some after-school activities, such as

- Dancing to his favorite music
- Spending a few minutes with an exercise bike or treadmill (if you have either)
- Doing some chores that you assign him—from cleaning up his room to emptying the dishwasher
- Turning on a children's exercise video and working out for 30 minutes

Many children are more likely to play an exercise video if siblings can work out with them. They may simply find it more fun to participate in physical activity with someone else. If your child has brothers or sisters, get them involved as much as possible.

WHAT DOES YOUR CHILD'S SCHOOL OFFER?

When you were in school, was physical education (PE) or recess your favorite "class"?

In many US schools, things have changed. Primarily because of budget cuts, PE programs have been sacrificed. Most states no longer mandate that their public schools must offer PE. In some schools, PE classes are limited to once or twice a week, or they've been eliminated completely. Children are paying the price.

As we've emphasized in this chapter, physical activity is crucial to your child's health and the management of his weight. If your child's school district has reduced or eliminated PE programs, you need to let the district know that you want these classes back. Tell your child's school principal. Write a letter to the members of the local school board. If you and other parents raise your voices, it might make a difference.

Finding Time to Be Active

See if this scenario sounds familiar: Your child has come home from school with 2 hours of homework, including studying for a math test the following day. He also needs to start working on a science fair project. And don't forget the clarinet lesson that's on his calendar as well. There seems to be barely enough time to fit in dinner and a bath or shower.

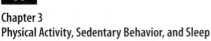

No wonder some kids feel that they just don't have time for physical activity. Their schedules are overflowing, and when they're overbooked, it's easy for physical activity to fall by the wayside.

As a parent, you need to intervene to make sure your child has time for all things that are important, and physical activity needs to be a priority.

Sit down with your child and help him structure his time after school so he can fit in everything that's most essential. For example, in planning the following day, you might say something like, "You have a block of after-school time tomorrow. Maybe that time isn't the best moment for homework, because it will take up the daylight hours when you could be outside playing. Why don't you think about choosing to play outdoors for 30 minutes or an hour after you get home? Then we'll go to your music lesson, and once you've eaten dinner and it's dark outside, you can do your homework. The evening is the time when you used to watch TV anyway, so it's a good time to get your homework done; watch TV or use the computer only if there is still time before bedtime. Remember to turn off the TV 30 minutes to an hour before bedtime so your screen time won't interfere with your sleep. And let's think about rescheduling your music lessons for the weekends."

As a parent, you can help your child find the opportunities to be active. If you're creative, the time will almost always be there.

Turning Family Time Into Active Time

For a lot of families, weekend afternoons are a time to be together at the movies or the mall. As enjoyable as those outings may be, start thinking about spending some of that family time doing physical activities that all of you like. Make special time for the family on a regular basis and try to make it physically active (and something not compatible with eating), such as going to the park for a hike, spending time gardening, or going to the zoo.

Some children are so averse to exercising that the first step in the right direction needs to be taken with their families. They may feel much more comfortable being active with their parents and siblings than with their peers, at least to start with. So why not play catch in the backyard, or dust off the tennis rackets in the closet and spend an hour hitting a tennis ball at the neighborhood courts? Rather than going to the movies, take a family hike in the hills near your home. When the whole family is involved, your child is more likely to join in. Once he starts losing weight and gets more accustomed to moving his body, he may feel less self-conscious and be more willing to step out and join a swimming program at the YMCA or take karate lessons at the local martial arts studio.

Spend a few moments thinking of other activities that your entire family can do together. Remember, the activity should be fun. If you need some suggestions, why not consider the following activities?

- Go to the park and throw the football back and forth.
- Play tag in the front yard.
- Organize a scavenger hunt.
- Go for a walk or walk the family dog together.
- Go to the community pool for a family swim.
- Buy a kite, put it together as a family activity, and fly it in the park. While you hold onto the kite string, let your child run with the kite until the wind catches it and sends it aloft.
- Take a family bike ride.
- Go horseback riding.
- Wash the car as a family activity.
- Go to the mall—walk from one end of the mall to the other, checking things out in the windows and shopping as needed.
- During the holiday season, take a family walk in the evening around the neighborhood and enjoy the holiday lights on the homes.

When you join in, your child will see that you believe physical activity is important, and you'll become his most important role model.

Other things to consider in everyday activities is walking up the stairs at stores or parking at a distance so you can walk. All these activities of daily living help keep your child and your family moving.

Screen Time: What's a Parent to Do?

We have all noticed how much screens have become part of our lives. From TV, to computers for homework and games, to tablets and cell phones, screens are everywhere and seem to be on all the time. Have you noticed families out to eat with everyone looking at their screens? How many times have you had to try to pull your child away from a computer game to come to the table or finish his homework?

Studies show that increased TV viewing is linked with obesity. More TV watching in childhood predicts obesity as an adult, and even in childhood, more hours of TV watched as a toddler increases the risk of obesity by age 7 years. Televisions now seem to be fixtures in children's bedrooms and result in more TV watching and less sleep, while in teens they are associated with a less healthy diet and fewer family meals.

Shifting the Balance

Screen time shifts the balance of healthy physical activity with little to no benefits. As we discussed with physical activity, children need to be active to become fit and maintain a healthy weight. And to no one's surprise, being active takes time, and in the busy life of a child and family, time for staying healthy is at a premium. When you think of the time children spend watching TV, playing video games, or staring at their phones, it may seem like you are trying to move a mountain to get them to do anything else. But you can shift the balance! Here are some tips to get started.

- Have each family member come up with their answer to the question, "What could you do if you didn't have your TV, computer, phone, etc, for an hour each day?"
- Then try setting a screen-free hour (or half-hour if an hour seems too much at first), where all screens are off in the house, and have family members report back on what they did.
- Try scheduling a family activity right after dinner, such as playing a game or listening to an audio book, instead of returning to screen time.
- Have TVs and phones turned off during mealtimes.
- Turn off the TV if no one is watching.

When Television Takes Control

Have you ever noticed that you suddenly develop a craving for pizza while watching TV or can't stop thinking about how good a nice cold soda would taste, or taken your children to the market and listened to them beg for a sugary cereal? Your TV is talking to you, and if numbers of commercials are any indication, it is telling you and your family to eat fast food, sugary cereals, and soft drinks. Games on the Internet, phone apps, and fast-food coupons delivered to phones are other ways unhealthy food messages are getting to your children. Children get the message, and that is when you find yourself in the grocery store with your child, who insists on foods advertised with his favorite characters on the box. Even movie previews depict unhealthy food habits and choices, let alone the array of options at the movie theater snack counter. So how do you get your voice heard over the media? Here are some ways to get started.

- Limit TV and find movies and shows without advertising for your children to watch.
- Talk about what you will buy before you go to the store; go with a list and stick to it.
- Stop before you get to the checkout lane and see if any sugary or snack foods have snuck into the cart.

- Talk about advertising with your children, what it means, and what you have decided to eat to keep your family healthy.
- Teens can be especially receptive to a discussion about how advertising is trying to change their behavior.

The Importance of Sleep

No one would argue that we would all like more sleep. In fact, when you look at recommended amounts of sleep per day, you wonder if anyone is getting enough sleep.

- Birth to 4 months: 14 to 15 hours (including naps)
- 4 to 12 months: 12 to 16 hours (including naps)
- 1 to 2 years: 11 to 14 hours (including naps)
- 3 to 5 years: 10 to 13 hours (including naps)
- 6 to 12 years: 9 to 12 hours
- 13 to 18 years: 8 to 10 hours

Lack of sleep increases the risk for obesity. Even getting as little as an extra hour of sleep per night can reduce the risk for obesity in a child younger than 10 years by 9%. Lack of sleep has been associated with increases in waist circumference, blood pressure, high-density lipo-protein cholesterol, and insulin resistance. The length of time a child sleeps is clearly important, but so is the quality of their sleep. In a child with obesity, sleep apnea, a common obesity-related condition, can drastically reduce the quality of sleep and is associated with increased risk of high blood pressure, bed-wetting, poor concentration in school, and daytime napping. This is something your pediatrician should check for. Good sleep habits start early, and here are some tips to help you get your child on the right track.

- Make sure your child has a bedtime routine. Giving a bath, reading a book, singing songs, and tucking your child in can all be part of what you do every night to pave the way to a good night's sleep.

- Keep track of when your child goes to sleep and gets up. Most parents, when asked, overestimate the amount of time their child sleeps.
- Minimize changes in bedtime and wake-up time by helping school-aged children and adolescents schedule homework time earlier in the afternoon or evening, limiting late-night screen time, and encouraging them to use study periods in school wisely. Many teens stay up late on school nights, and then have to get up early for school, and they make up the difference on the weekends by sleeping late. This change in sleep pattern has been associated with obesity.
- Keep screens out of the bedroom. Television watching and phone interaction interfere with sleep, and limiting screen use to up to 30 minutes before bedtime may help your child settle down.
- Check with your pediatrician about sleep apnea. Children with obesity are more prone to have sleep apnea, and snoring, restless sleeping, sleeping on multiple pillows, or sitting up can all be signs of sleep apnea, as can daytime napping, bed-wetting, and doing poorly in school. Your pediatrician can help diagnose and treat sleep apnea.

Looking Forward

In the months and years ahead, don't back away from your commitment to promote physical activity in your child's life. Encourage any form of exercise or other activity that he enjoys and is willing to do regularly. Not only will he be better able to successfully manage his weight, but he has a much greater likelihood of enjoying a healthy life well into and throughout adulthood.

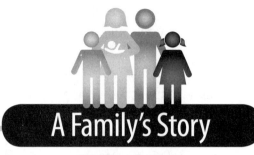

A Family's Story

The Appointment

Jerry's appointment with his pediatrician came quickly, and the whole family went to the visit with Dr Scott. Jean brought the letter from the school and Dr Scott reviewed it, checked Jerry's height and weight, and asked some questions about the family's nutrition and activity. Jean was prepared for the nutrition questions—in fact, she had started writing down what Jerry ate—but the answers to the physical activity questions surprised her and Bob. They realized that it had been quite some time since Jerry had gone out to play in the backyard after school. These days he was fascinated with his new video game, and when his friends came over, they all stayed inside. Bob hadn't realized that physical education was only once a week and that Jerry's favorite activity at recess was talking with his friends about their favorite superheroes instead of playing an active game. The pediatrician asked Jerry what he watched on TV, and Jerry was able to rattle off show after show. Dr Scott then asked him, "What could you do if you didn't watch TV?" and Jerry had a tough time coming up with an answer. With all of this in mind, Jean and Bob began to think about planning a family activity for the weekend, and Jerry piped up that he thought he might like to go the park some days after school to play basketball with some of his friends.

Key Points to Remember

 As you plan to help your child increase his physical activity, check in with your child's pediatrician for guidance on amount and type and to make sure your child is physically ready for the exercise he chooses. The AAP recommends 1 hour or more of physical activity per day.

 Children with special health care needs can participate in many sports and activities, so talk with your child's pediatrician about what accommodations your child may need and what opportunities exist for him to participate.

 Time can often seem to be a limiting factor when trying to work physical activity into a routine. Work on an after-school and weekend routine with your child that builds in time to be active.

 Explore after-school and community programs as ways of helping your child increase his activity.

 Make family time more active—a walk after dinner, a game of catch on the weekends, or a trip to the park.

Resources

American Academy of Pediatrics Council on Sports Medicine and Fitness and Council on School Health. Active healthy living: prevention of childhood obesity through increased physical activity. *Pediatrics*. 2006;117(5):1834–1842

Beccuti G, Pannain S. Sleep and obesity. *Curr Opin Clin Nutr Metab Care*. 2011;14(4):402–412

Hakim F, Kheirandish-Gozal L, Gozal D. Obesity and altered sleep: a pathway to metabolic derangements in children? *Semin Pediatr Neurol*. 2015;22(2):77–85

Miller AL, Lumeng JC, LeBourgeois MK. Sleep patterns and obesity in childhood. *Curr Opin Endocrinol Diabetes Obes*. 2015;22(1):41–47

National Physical Activity Plan Alliance. 2016 US Report Card on Physical Activity for Children and Youth. http://www.physicalactivityplan.org/projects/reportcard.html. Accessed October 30, 2017

Pagani LS, Fitzpatrick C, Barnett TA, Dubow E. Prospective associations between early childhood television exposure and academic, psychosocial, and physical well-being by middle childhood. *Arch Pediatr Adolesc Med*. 2010;164(5):425–431

Chapter 4

Your Role as a Parent: Developing a Consistent Approach

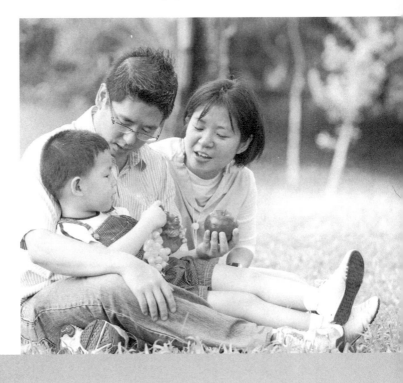

Parenting is filled with challenges. As your child grows from infancy through childhood and adolescence, there is no one more important to her development than you. Not a day goes by when you're not called on to ensure her physical, emotional, social, and intellectual well-being.

If your child is overweight or has obesity, however, you may feel that your parenting responsibilities have been turned up a notch. Almost by definition, weight management is a difficult challenge. As the primary person keeping your child consistently moving in the direction of a healthy weight—one meal or snack after another, one physical activity after the next—your challenges may seem daunting at times.

In this and the next 2 chapters, we'll equip you with information to help take much of the anxiety out of your parenting role. In the months and years ahead, the most important changes will start and continue at home with your family and child. We'll examine how your own parenting style may influence your child's success in her efforts at controlling her weight. You'll also find some concrete parenting guidance to help your child navigate the inevitable obstacles she'll encounter as she makes progress toward her goals. Chapters 9 through 12 include a section about the parent's role, featuring action items, strategies, and tips that highlight what you can do to further help your child in maintaining a healthy weight at that specific age.

Parents often say that they have difficulty keeping their children's eating and activity behaviors pointed in the right direction. Sometimes, they may believe that they just don't have the skills to keep their family consistently on track. They simply might feel weary about making decisions, on almost an hour-by-hour basis, that can help their children achieve a healthy weight. They might also find it difficult to deal with their children's complaints that they are no longer able to eat all the foods they want when they want, or that they are miserable because they can't watch television (TV) all day on Saturday anymore. No wonder parents can feel exhausted.

Putting Health First

Do these scenarios sound familiar? Do you sometimes feel overwhelmed by the responsibilities of parenting a child struggling with weight? Do you often feel that you're not up to the task, or does your child somehow make you feel heartless and mean-spirited when you insist on refocusing the family in a way that supports the loss of her excess weight?

The good news is that because you are reading this book you have made a commitment to a healthier child and family. Keep in mind that nearly every parent of a child with obesity feels discouraged from time to time. But don't lose your direction. It is important to keep thinking of your decisions to move in a healthy direction as more than weight-related decisions. Every decision you make about healthy eating and activity, screen time, and sleeping is a health decision, and remember that improving your child's health is your ultimate goal. After all, as a parent, you're used to making other kinds of health decisions for your family. You do it every day, and it's something that you've become very good at. For example, you don't have a problem making sure that your child gets all the vaccinations she needs, even when she complains that she doesn't want a shot today. If your 12-year-old were to tell you that one of the kids in the neighborhood is smoking cigarettes and she wants to try it, too, you wouldn't hesitate to say "no" in the most forceful way possible. Your child's health is a priority, and it's an area in which you've been making decisions without hesitation. As your child gets older you will have different kinds of discussions about the positives and negatives of her health choices and focusing on the skills she will need to make these healthy choices for herself.

Remember, obesity is a threat to her health, increasing her risk of developing a long list of serious illnesses. She is more likely to have high blood pressure. She may become vulnerable to type 2 diabetes. Blood tests might show that she has elevated triglyceride levels or a problem with her liver. She could develop asthma or gallstones.

For these reasons, you shouldn't think twice about doing what it takes to get your child's problem with weight under control. As her parent, you're the protector of her well-being. It's one of your most important responsibilities. Each time you make a weight-related decision, it's as important as any other judgment about your family's health. You can't be passive when your child's health is at stake. By making the right decisions now, you'll be affecting her well-being far into the future.

You Are the Agent for Change

Your child's efforts to lose weight are like a journey. At times, it might seem like the journey is taking you and your child down a long and winding road where the results you're seeking are far off in the distance. As an adult and a parent, you are the person who needs to make sure that your child and entire family stay the course. You are the captain of the ship that is helping your child navigate and surmount all the challenges that are ahead. *You are the agent for change and role model for healthy decision-making that can guide your child's own decision-making as she grows into an independent adult.*

As you guide your child along the path toward a healthier weight, you need to stay a step ahead of her to keep her moving toward the destination. That means focusing some of your energy on establishing routines and guidelines that set the stage for her success. This should be a familiar parental task because, in one form or another, you've been doing it since your child was an infant. In the preschool years, for example, you taught her rules for negotiating her way successfully through the world she lives in—the importance of crossing streets only when the traffic signal is green, sharing toys with friends, and brushing her teeth before she goes to sleep. In the same way, you need to create routines and guidelines that will help her make healthy choices today.

Where should you begin? A good starting point is right at home. That means taking charge of the family's day-to-day environment. It means creating the conditions for change to take place, with minimal conflict or confrontation. It means eliminating as many temptations as possible.

In the previous chapters, we've already given you some ideas for seizing control of what goes on at home, from keeping unhealthy snacks out of the cupboard to taking the entire family on a walk after dinner rather than turning on the TV. It also means giving your child choices but only within the limits of safe, healthy boundaries. For instance

- You can provide the play equipment, and she can decide whether to jump rope or throw a ball against the garage door.
- You can invite her to help prepare her lunch and let her choose from among several healthy entrées that you can make together.
- You can keep tempting high-calorie snack foods (like cookies and candy bars) out of your grocery cart and, instead, let her choose from among healthier alternatives to stock your kitchen cupboard.

Remember, your home environment is something that you can control almost completely. It gives you enormous power in becoming an agent for change and helping her successfully manage her obesity.

Customizing Approaches for Your Family

No two families are alike. What works for yours may send another family spinning out of control, even when they're dealing with the exact same issues. There is no single best way of managing a particular situation, so be willing to fine-tune the strategies you adopt until you're getting the job done.

Of course, you need to identify the changes you want and what may be getting in the way of those changes being made, particularly over the long term. If your child overdoes the afternoon snacking when she gets home from school, maybe you need to limit the time she has available for indulging in these munchies in addition to providing and maintaining the healthiest possible nutritional environment at home. Keep her attention directed elsewhere, perhaps by having her play outside with friends immediately after school or getting her involved in an after-school activity.

Not surprisingly, your parental interventions will evolve as your child gets older. You can't expect the same approaches that worked when she was 8 years old to still work at 14 years. As a teenager, if she'd prefer to sit at the computer for hours after school, exchanging instant messages with her friends and eating all the while, you're not going to necessarily be able to send her outside to the neighborhood playground with swings and monkey bars. But you can explore other activities that will keep her busy. How about encouraging your adolescent to volunteer at the public library by helping out at the preschoolers' story hour? Or encourage her to sign up for an ice-skating class or tennis lessons? Or maybe she can try out for the school softball team. In virtually every community, there are plenty of healthy after-school options.

Whatever your child decides to do, you will want to monitor the situation consistently. Many parents assume that once their children reach a certain age, they'll know what to do to stay active, or they'll instinctively choose a healthier snack over a less healthy one. Not true. Every child can use some help and support. For that reason, don't leave these decisions solely in your child's hands. You're still the parent, and you're a full partner in this change that your child is making. It's your parental responsibility to make sure she keeps moving in the direction of better health.

SETTING SHORT-TERM, ACHIEVABLE GOALS

If your child is determined to lose weight, have the two of you (along with your child's pediatrician) discussed a weight-loss strategy? No matter how ambitious the goal, it's important that you encourage her to set some short-term goals that she can reach along the way that will keep her motivated to stay the course.

Use this same approach in every aspect of this program. Guide your child toward deciding what she wants to achieve, and then help her get there in small steps. If she needs to spend more time being physically active, perhaps start with just a few minutes of outdoor play after school and build on that.

See yourself as a parental support system. Help your child set short-term goals and make small changes that can add up to big improvements. If those goals involve reducing her time in front of the TV and becoming more physically active, they'll become an important way for the entire family to move a step closer to a healthier lifestyle.

The Power of Family

Imagine your child sitting on the couch along with the entire family, watching a movie. But while everyone else is munching on cookies in front of the TV, she's trying to restrain herself from reaching for a handful of her own. It's a bit of torture that is setting her up for failure.

Without a doubt, it is much easier to make changes when those around you are adopting the same new behaviors as you. As we'll emphasize throughout this book, your child's success in achieving a healthy weight is dependent on the support of the entire family—parents, partners, siblings, grandparents, uncles, aunts, cousins, and anyone else who spends time with her. Part of your parenting responsibility is to let the other adults in your child's life (like schoolteachers, church leaders, scoutmasters, and relatives) know about your child's efforts so they won't undermine them. All it takes are a few acts of sabotage, however innocent or unintentional, to tip your child in the wrong direction and derail weeks of her best effort.

At every opportunity, your family needs to demonstrate support for your child. You need to be consistent in approaching your child's struggle with obesity because you have the primary responsibility for managing her nutrition, physical activity, screen time, and sleep. If you're separated or divorced from your child's other parent, it is important to try to share information with your former spouse on an ongoing basis and to work toward mutually deciding on any changes in the environment that need to be made at each of your respective homes.

Structured Eating

As you might guess, when you have a child trying to lose weight, you need to pay particular attention to mealtimes. They should be firmly structured not only for your child but for the entire family. In general, 3 meals and 1 to 2 snacks per day, without any meal skipping, are optimal (if your child skips a meal, she'll become over-hungry and set herself up for overeating). Also, if she knows that dinner is going to be served at 6:00 pm, she'll be less likely to start searching for a snack at 5:30 pm, whereas if dinner is served at a different time every night (for example, sometimes at 6:00 pm, but other times at 8:00 pm), she might grab a snack at 5:30 pm rather than risk having to wait 2 or 3 hours for her hunger pangs to be satisfied.

There's another very important element to structured eating, and that's ensuring that the family eats together as often as possible with no distractions. In too many homes, families rarely sit down for a meal together, and when they do, the TV or the screens are on and no one (except maybe for a sitcom star or the local newscaster) says a word throughout the dinner hour. Screens are a disruption that you should avoid while you're eating.

Just how important are family meals? In many households, they're the only period of the day when the family is together, giving every adult and child an opportunity to talk about what happened at school or work. It's a time when the family can grow closer to one another. It's also a time to teach your child about healthy, balanced meals and appropriate portion sizes and when you can serve as a role model for healthy eating. You can also offer encouragement to your child, celebrate her successes, and reassure her if she's having difficulties. As an added benefit, you'll be able to keep an eye on what and how much she is eating.

One other note: These family meals will probably become less common as your child enters adolescence. Once she's involved in rehearsals for the high school play or is gone because of a part-time job at the local pharmacy, you'll covet those days when the family could be together at the dinner table. Treat these opportunities as precious moments that will become some of your sweetest family memories many years down the road.

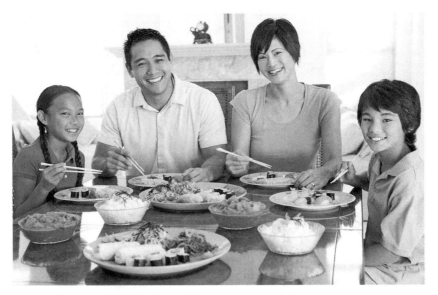

WEEKEND PERILS

Some parents feel they've got a good grip on how their children's lives unfold during the week. There's a structure to the day, Monday through Friday, incorporating school and extracurricular activities, that helps them effectively manage their children's nutrition and activity levels.

Then the weekend arrives. The routine that they relied on during the previous 5 days simply isn't there, and that's when trouble often rises to the surface. On Saturdays, the kids might end up watching TV from sunup to exhaustion (if you let them). In the process, they're not getting any exercise, and they're probably overindulging on snacks when they're not playing with the remote control. Then there are the weekend dinners at the family's favorite all-you-can-eat restaurant, or the afternoon at the baseball stadium where everyone has one hot dog too many.

What's the solution? Saturdays and Sundays need to be planned as carefully as the rest of your child's week. Help schedule her time so that at least part of every Saturday and Sunday is devoted to physical activity. Sign her up for a Saturday afternoon sports program at the community center. At home, make sure that only healthy snacks are available for her to grab. There's no need for your child to backslide on the weekends, but it will take some consistent parental planning to ensure that it doesn't happen.

Partnering With Your Child's Pediatrician

Since the time your child was born, you have relied on her pediatrician to play multiple roles in your child's life, from providing physical examinations to treating her illnesses to administering her immunizations on schedule. Don't overlook the important supportive role your pediatrician can play by partnering with your family in helping your child achieve a healthy weight.

Each time you visit the pediatrician's office, particularly for scheduled checkups, your doctor or a nurse will weigh and measure your child and calculate her body mass index. He or she will check your child's overall health status and monitor any obesity-related health conditions she may have, such as high blood pressure or high cholesterol levels.

Your pediatrician can also talk with your child about her weight problem at a level appropriate for her age. The doctor can help you and your child prioritize the changes that need to be made first to get her weight under control and help you set some health goals, including lifestyle changes such as eating more healthfully, becoming more physically active, and watching less TV.

Also, turn to your child's pediatrician for guidance on child development issues. The doctor can answer questions like, "At my child's age, what is she capable of doing on her own as we're adopting a more healthful lifestyle?" As you might guess, and your pediatrician can help explain, a 14-year-old is able to do much more than a 4-year-old. It isn't developmentally appropriate, for example, to put your 4-year-old in charge of getting her own snacks from the refrigerator and expect her to make appropriate choices, but a 14-year-old who you've educated about healthy snacking might be trusted to do so.

THE COMMUNITY AND SCHOOLS

Your parenting responsibilities extend far beyond what's happening in your home. Your child spends plenty of time at school and perhaps a child care setting, and as we've emphasized elsewhere in this book, you need to make sure that the foods and beverages she eats are healthy and compatible with the nutritional plan that she's following at home. In chapters 2 and 3, we emphasized the importance of gathering information about school menus, learning what your child is being fed at child care, and asking how much physical activity she's getting. If you're not pleased with the answers you're getting—perhaps your child's school has phased out recess or serves too many high-fat, high-calorie foods and snacks without much nutritional value in the cafeteria or student store—you need to raise your voice and request changes. If your child is in preschool, talk with the teachers and ask for healthier snacks. You might find that your child's teacher will actively become an ally in supporting your child's efforts to achieve a healthy weight.

Recruit other parents to join you and raise your voices in unison. In the best-case scenario, your school administrators will reassess what they're doing and make changes toward better nutrition for the entire school. If change isn't forthcoming, start packing a lunch for your child to ensure that she'll get the kind of healthy nourishment she needs.

Keeping Focused on the Goal

Particularly in a book about children struggling with weight, it might be easy to become preoccupied with the kinds and amounts of food that your child eats. Of course, we're not saying that your child's nutrition isn't important—in fact, we devoted Chapter 2 to it. Even so, there are other significant topics that deserve your attention as well.

Much of your focus as a parent should be on changing your child's behavior and lifestyle. It should be on consistently living a *healthier* life. As we'll emphasize throughout this book, the weight will come off if you and your child are making healthy choices. And if you are struggling, the sections on troubleshooting and help from your pediatrician can help get you and your child back on track. Once you let go of your preoccupation with your child's weight and incorporate healthy eating, physical activity, and better sleeping habits into her routine, it will free you to handle what needs to be done to ensure her overall good health.

Remember, you and your child are on a journey that, like any trip, requires a plan and clear vision of your destination. Remind her that you and your family are on this journey toward better health together, every step of the way, and you are preparing your child for a life of healthy decision-making.

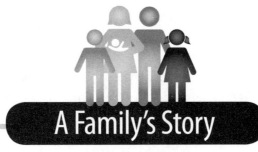

A Family's Story

Becoming a Team

Jean and Bob were on their way to making healthy changes for their family. But they quickly realized that they needed to have an approach to pull everyone together. They decided after the visit with Dr Scott to

- Plan a family activity that involved physical activity on the weekend.

- Cut down from 2 to 1 fast-food meal per week.

- Have a family screen time schedule.

Everyone loved going to the zoo on Saturday as the family activity, so Jerry and Melissa began thinking up more family activities, like going to the state park, bowling, and playing a family game of basketball. Cutting back on fast food was harder. Melissa thought that it wasn't fair for her to have to cut back, since it was Jerry who needed to lose weight. Jerry missed his TV shows. Jean and Bob sat down with the family and explained that the changes they all were making were to get the whole family healthier. They said they knew it wasn't always easy but were proud of Jerry and Melissa for trying to stay with the plan and encouraged them to be a part of these changes as much as possible by having them suggest healthy meal options and fun activities that would make everyone happy and more willing to participate.

Chapter 5

What's Your Parenting Style?
Assessing Your Strengths
and Challenges

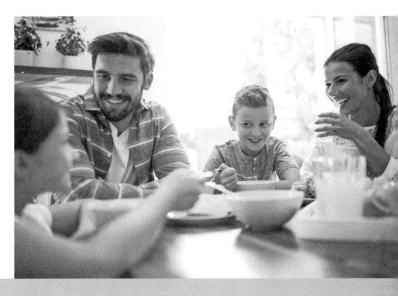

If your child is going to succeed at achieving a healthy weight, that effort needs to begin at home. The way your child eats starts right in your own kitchen. The choices he makes to become active may begin with a conversation over the dinner table and lead to the parks and playgrounds in your own neighborhood.

In these parenting chapters, you'll learn that your skills, style, and decisions as a parent clearly matter where your child's weight is concerned. At the same time, for most parents, even those who are (or once had been) overweight or had obesity themselves, this may still seem like largely uncharted territory. After all, helping a child reach his healthy weight and fully understanding the parent–child dynamics that can contribute to his success or setbacks aren't taught in most parenting books and classes. In this chapter and the one that follows, we'll help you examine and more fully appreciate how you and the entire family contribute to your child's ability to achieve a healthy weight. As you'll read, you can help him see the importance of adopting healthy habits that can last a lifetime. On the other hand, you might realize that you have been using food in a negative way (as a reward, for example) that could undermine your child's hope of successful weight loss. We'll even explore how your own childhood experiences, including the messages you got from your own parents about food and weight, may be a factor in how you and your child relate to each other about this issue.

As we'll emphasize throughout this book, a balanced diet and regular physical activity can promote good health in your child. Meaningful change will happen only if you're willing to work with him on taking small steps forward that can make a big difference in his well-being and weight. The most powerful changes occur when parents and families make the same changes themselves on this journey to help their children lead healthier lifestyles.

Chapter 5
What's Your Parenting Style? Assessing Your Strengths and Challenges

Your Family Background

Understanding yourself as a parent starts with looking at your own family when you were growing up. Parents often react to their own childhood experiences by either trying to reproduce them or trying not to make the same mistakes. Either way, it is important to know where you came from to plan where you are going.

Let's begin by examining your own childhood and the relationship that you've had to food and body weight. By answering the following questions thoughtfully, you may gain some insights into your current thinking about your child's food intake and his obesity.

You (and your spouse or your child's other parent) should consider these questions and talk through your answers together. You might find some similarities in your backgrounds—or some marked differences that could contribute to conflicts or problems in the way each of you approaches your child's excess weight.

- When you were growing up, did your family life tend to revolve around food and meals?
  - What about at family gatherings and holidays?
- At mealtimes, was there always plenty of food on the dining room table?
- Did your parent(s) place serving dishes on the dinner table so you could easily help yourself to seconds and choose your own portion sizes?
  - Did you often take seconds?
- Did your parent(s) usually insist that you eat everything on your plate, even when you were no longer hungry?
- Were you overweight or did you have obesity as a child?
  - If "yes," do you think your excess weight changed your life in any major way? If so, how?

- Did you often try to lose weight as a child?
  - Were those efforts successful?
  - Were they ever a source of conflict between you and your parents?
- Did your mother and/or father have overweight or obesity?
- Did your grandparents have overweight or obesity?
- As a child, were you often preoccupied with thoughts of food during the day?
- Did you eat secretly so your parent(s) and other family members wouldn't know how much you ate?
  - If "yes," how often did you eat this way (for example, daily, weekly)?
- During your childhood, did your parent(s) sometimes use food as
  - A reward?
  - A bribe?
  - A source of comfort?
- Were you physically active with regularity as a child?
  - In school?
  - Outside of school?
  - In youth sports (for example, soccer, Little League)?
- What types of activities did you participate in?
- Did your family participate in physical activities together?
- What types of physical activities did you do as a family?
- If you could change anything about your childhood (as it relates to the issues mentioned here), what would you change?
- How do you think your own childhood experiences with food and physical activity influence the way you're raising your own child today?

Did some of these questions strike a chord with you? In many cultures, for example, food is a very important part of family life. When extended families get together, much of the attention seems to focus on large, high-calorie meals, and as a result, the waistlines of everyone at the dinner table often pay the price.

Chapter 5
What's Your Parenting Style? Assessing Your Strengths and Challenges

On the other hand, perhaps you grew up in a family for which money was scarce and there wasn't a lot of extra food for second helpings—or sometimes even first helpings! These are experiences that will linger with you for a lifetime, and when you have children of your own, you might think, "It's important for me to make sure my children will always have *all* the food they want."

As you contemplate the answers to these previous questions, think back to your family's health history, including whether you, your spouse or your child's other parent, or other family members have had obesity-related chronic health problems over the years, including heart disease, high cholesterol levels, diabetes, and asthma. These medical histories can provide clues to your own child's risks and should motivate you to work hard to help your child achieve a healthy weight, which reduces his likelihood of developing chronic illnesses now and in the future.

Use the answers to these questions as a springboard for family discussion, and help everyone understand what may be driving some of your own concerns about your child's weight and how you're trying to deal with them. Maybe you grew up with parents who told you to eat everything on your plate, perhaps using the logic that there were "children starving in <a foreign country>." As an adult, you know the perils of prompting your child to continue eating even after he's full; if you do it routinely, it can deliver a knockout to all your positive efforts at encouraging weight loss. By sharing the experiences of your own childhood, you may better understand some of the issues that have arisen in your family life today.

PUTTING FOOD IN PERSPECTIVE

As important as it is to pay attention to the dietary and lifestyle changes that can help your child successfully manage his weight, don't overfocus on them, particularly your child's food choices.

If you struggled with overweight yourself when you were his age, you might feel that you'll do whatever it takes to help him avoid the same emotional pain that you went through. But some parents become obsessed with the food their children are consuming. They spend most of their mealtimes together—and just about every other available moment—talking with their children about what they're eating or shouldn't be eating. They discuss calories, portion sizes, and fat content. They focus on the latest news about fad diets. You'd think there was nothing else going on in their children's worlds.

There is such an overemphasis on food in some families that it gets in the way of having a balanced relationship between parents and children. Remember, there's more to your child's life than what he's eating and how much he weighs. (How about asking, "What did you do at school today?" or "How much homework do you have tonight?") By keeping food in perspective and focusing on the rest of your child's interests and activities, you can make mealtime a positive time for both of you.

Family Interactions

The support your child needs to steadily and successfully lose weight should be a family affair. As you've read in earlier chapters, your child needs the entire family to get on board—parents, grandparents, brothers, and sisters—and unanimously agree to keep foods like potato chips and chocolate chip cookies out of the house and get more physical activity, even among those who have no excess weight to lose.

Keep in mind that as a parent, you want *all* your children to live a life of optimal health, no matter what their weights. You want their hearts to stay healthy. You want their blood pressure to stay normal. You want them to avoid diabetes. For that reason, this is an important and even exciting journey for the family to embark on, and although you're the tour guide on this trip, it's one that the whole family needs to take

90

Chapter 5
What's Your Parenting Style? Assessing Your Strengths and Challenges

together. Everyone should sign on as a demonstration of support for your child struggling with weight—and in the process, they'll improve their own well-being.

Over the ensuing weeks and months, it is helpful if you have regular family meetings. This is a time to discuss how everyone is doing on this mission to better health. What has been the hardest part for everyone? What was the most difficult change to make, and what was easier than anyone had imagined? Are all family members on board with these changes? What still needs to be done? Also, make sure that the family understands that almost inevitably, there will be ups and downs in this journey.

At times, an older child may feel guilty if he plateaus and seems to be getting nowhere in his weight-loss efforts, or perhaps he'll regain some of the weight he had lost. He might even become the target of blame or anger from siblings who feel he hasn't been trying hard enough. Explain that pointing fingers only gets in the way of progress. As long as there's internal bickering and family members who are playing the blame game, it's virtually impossible for your child to move forward again. This is a time to reemphasize how important family support is to every family member, whether they are trying to manage their weight, become a better student, or improve their skills at sports. Rooting for each other, using positive language, and celebrating success is at the heart of family support.

DIVORCE AND DIFFERING OPINIONS

If you and your child's other parent are divorced or separated, it is important that both of you work extra hard to make sure you remain active players in your child's support team. Take responsibility for maintaining the healthiest possible home environment. Make sure it's as conducive as possible to helping your child reach his weight-loss goals.

Even if you and your child's other parent don't see eye to eye on everything, your child's well-being should be an area where you can come together. Nevertheless, getting both parents and other family members to participate actively in a child's weight-loss program doesn't always happen. In some families, only one parent recognizes that the child's weight is a problem; the other parent, particularly if this parent never had a weight problem of his or her own, might have a "What's the big deal?" attitude and may not understand how hard it can be to lose weight. If this is an issue in your family, working with your pediatrician can take this into consideration and help you navigate a healthy lifestyle plan.

Emotions and Food

Children (as well as adults) use food for reasons other than to satisfy their hunger and nutritional needs. In fact, children who have obesity often may eat in response to their emotions and feelings. For example, at the beginning of this chapter, we raised the issue of whether your own parents used food for comfort in your household. This is a common phenomenon, beginning at birth. If a baby's crying or irritability is typically met with human (breast) milk or infant formula, feeding may become a way of calming and quieting him. At birthdays and holidays, when children are surrounded by family and are feeling loved, they're often given cookies or other desserts that become a symbol of this love and caring.

It may be that whenever your own child is feeling anxious, perhaps related to an upcoming math test or because he's being teased at school, he may turn back to food as one way of making him feel better. At the same time, however, there are many other reasons beyond comfort that

92

Chapter 5
What's Your Parenting Style? Assessing Your Strengths and Challenges

may prompt children to eat. For example, does your child sometimes reach for food when he's experiencing any of these feelings?

- Boredom
- Depression
- Stress
- Frustration

- Insecurity
- Loneliness
- Fatigue
- Resentment

- Anger
- Happiness

Even though food can become a welcome companion for your child, the outcome may not be quite what he expected. Ironically, if he overeats to soften feelings of insecurity or depression, for instance, or perhaps because of stress over an oral report he needs to give at school, he may feel even worse after a food binge, knowing that it can aggravate his weight problem. Before the food is even digested, he might be feeling guilt or shame.

In fact, one of your biggest parenting challenges is for you and your child to determine whether he's eating for the right reasons. Ask yourself questions like, does he eat at times other than regular mealtimes and snacks? Is he munching at every opportunity? What factors might be contributing to his overeating that call for you to intervene?

Some parents inadvertently contribute to their children's weight by rewarding their children with food (does an A on a test sometimes lead to a trip to the ice cream shop?). If this is the case, it is important to think about other, healthier ways to offer praise and rewards. For a young child, how about giving him a few stickers as a reward or perhaps schedule a shopping trip to buy a toy, a new pair of shoes, or a book? Spending time together can provide the positive energy for your child to accomplish his goals.

Don't overlook the importance of verbal praise. When your child is doing things right, tell him. Notice how words of approval for positive behavior can boost his self-esteem and help keep him motivated to continue making the right decisions for his health and weight. Even when he's having difficulties staying on course with his diet, look for other ways to offer praise ("You walked more than half a mile today; that's so great!"). When he backslides, don't nag him or make him feel like he failed. Encourage him to keep moving forward, and even if he complains from time to time ("I want a soft drink, not ice water!"), encourage him to stay the course. Offer him all the support he needs and deserves.

It's important for parents to listen to how they're speaking to their children. Is it mostly negative? Is it often critical? It's hard for anyone, including children, to make changes in that kind of environment. Some parents try to embarrass their children into making changes ("Billy, you're getting fatter again!"), figuring that if he sees himself as unsightly, he'll be motivated to lose weight. Don't count on that strategy working. Even if your child makes changes under these circumstances, those improvements are not likely to last without some parental praise and positive reinforcement along the way.

94

Chapter 5
What's Your Parenting Style? Assessing Your Strengths and Challenges

EQUAL VERSUS EQUALITY

The goals for diet and physical activity should be different for a 10-year-old than a 5-year-old, taking into account their different developmental stages, ages, and sizes. Your children, however, may not see it that way. At the dinner table, your 5-year-old daughter might say that she wants to eat the same amount of food as her older sister. You need to explain that their ages and stages are different. Yes, you will treat them with equality, but that doesn't mean that they'll receive equal portion sizes or that you'll challenge them to exercise in exactly the same way. Paying attention to each individual child's needs for rightsized nutrition and activity is more easily done at home than when you eat out.

That's why, when weight loss is a goal for one or more family members, consider eating most of your meals at home, where you'll have better control of the amounts of food that end up on everyone's plates. When the family eats dinner together, you can prepare the same foods for everyone, perhaps giving all the children servings of chicken, vegetables, and potatoes, along with a glass of milk. You shouldn't be serving your 8-year-old and 4-year-old the identical portion sizes, though. The portions on their plates should be age appropriate.

As we pointed out in Chapter 4, you'll also probably find that when the family sits down for a meal together, good things happen. According to the American Academy of Pediatrics, children who eat meals with their families are likely to consume more vegetables and fruits and less fried foods and soft drinks than children who eat less frequently with their families. It's another good reason to turn mealtime into family time.

Time for Reevaluation

Next, let's review the same questions we asked at the beginning of this chapter. Even though you've already thought about some of these topics in earlier chapters of this book (like questions about your child's eating habits and activity level), reemphasizing them here can help you more fully understand the family dynamics that contribute to your child's obesity and help you in the journey toward better health on which your family is embarking. You'll see what you're doing well and where you might need to improve.

No matter how you answer these questions, one thing is certain— you're reading this book because you care deeply about the well-being of your child. You want the best for him, including as healthy a life as possible. If there are moments when you or your child feels discouraged, don't give up. Move past those negative thoughts. Be patient. This is a long-term adventure; it was never designed as a quick fix or a rapid over-and-done process.

Continue to teach your family a healthier way of life. Keep making small changes and, over time, they'll make a big difference in your child's health. Remember, making reasonable changes is a reasonable thing to do where your child's health is concerned.

In the next chapter, we'll describe in detail some common trouble areas that you could encounter on this journey, from children who sneak food to cultural issues that can influence what your child eats. Chapter 6 will equip you with some tools and suggestions for continuing to move forward toward your child's weight-loss goals.

96

Chapter 5
What's Your Parenting Style? Assessing Your Strengths and Challenges

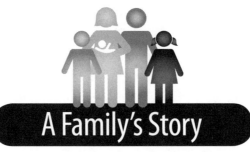

A Family's Story

The Grandparents Visit

Things were going well with the changes Jerry and his family were making. Family weekend activities were a big hit, and Jerry and Melissa had gotten used to their screen time schedule and eating out once instead of twice per week. But just when everyone was thinking about what other changes they might make, Grandma and Grandpa came for a visit. Jean explained to her parents that the whole family was working on adopting healthier habits and that the pediatrician was concerned about Jerry's weight. Both grandparents were surprised and said that Jerry was just big-boned like his uncles and that they weren't sure that Jean and Bob should be so concerned. Jean called a family meeting and asked the kids to share with their grandparents what the family was doing. Melissa started and said they were cooking more meals at home and she liked helping her mom make healthy food for dinner. Jerry said he enjoyed going places with his family on the weekends and looked forward to it all week.

Sitting everyone down and discussing some of the family changes helped Jerry and Melissa's grandparents see how these new habits were positively affecting the family physically and emotionally. It allowed them to get on board and join in on helping promote a healthy lifestyle while also having fun! That weekend the whole family went on a picnic by the lake, and Grandpa showed the children how to fish.

Key Points to Remember

 Your own relationship with food and weight, dating back to your childhood, can influence the way you parent your own child.

 Your child needs the support of your entire family. All family members should participate in the journey to better health.

 Provide your child with plenty of parental praise and positive reinforcement, but don't reward him with food.

 Finger-pointing gets in the way of progress toward weight loss and better health.

 Divorced or separated parents should both take responsibility for maintaining the healthiest possible environment in their own homes.

 Keep your child's weight problem in perspective. There's more to your relationship with him than the number on the bathroom scale.

Chapter 6

Parenting Challenges: Working With Your Child to Get Back to Good Health

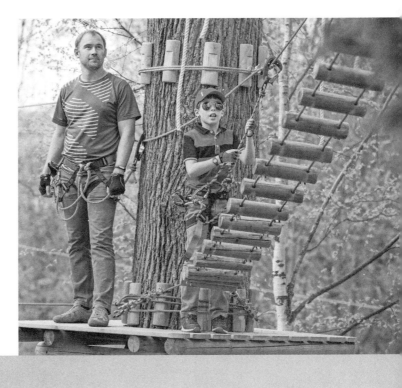

Even though you and your family may be fully committed to helping your child try new foods, eat more fruits and vegetables, try healthier snacks, and exercise more, many challenges can still arise on this journey. If you are thinking about helping your child with her weight but are not sure if you are ready to start, don't stop reading. Spending time to get prepared to make change is important. Continue reading, jot down thoughts and questions, and talk with other family members and your child's pediatrician to get support. In fact, it's unrealistic to think that problems won't develop that require your attention and action. But even though there may be obstacles along the way, you can succeed in helping your child and your family find the path to better health.

In this chapter, we'll describe some of the most common challenges that you're likely to encounter. You'll also read about other relevant issues that may apply to your child, from sneaking food to being teased and bullied. We'll examine ways you can intervene to keep your child moving forward. Sometimes, when setbacks happen, parents feel frustrated and may begin to bargain, cajole, and just plain focus on what's not happening with food and activity. This is tempting, but remember that your job is to provide good nutrition in proper portions to your child and family and then let them decide how much of that portion to eat and to encourage activity in a positive way. Staying positive and focusing on what's going right and all the other aspects of your child's life can help keep nutrition and activity change moving along.

Managing Setbacks and Detours

No matter how strong your child's determination is to gain better control over her food and activity choices, she'll probably experience some setbacks from time to time. Maybe she'll overeat for several days in a row. She might grab some unhealthy foods in the school cafeteria when she's feeling stressed about upcoming final examinations. Perhaps she'll attend a birthday party and help herself to more than one very large slice of cake—with extra ice cream on top.

As discouraged as you and your child might feel at those moments, you need to keep these lapses in perspective. You don't have to view them as the start down a slippery slope from which there's no turning back. Instead, think of them as just minor stumbling blocks, which is exactly what they are. Even if they add a pound or two to your child's weight, they're certainly not a reason for her to give up and abandon all the successes she's had so far. Remember that you are helping your child develop lifelong habits for healthy eating and activity. Learning how to make wise health decisions about nutrition and activity is what's important. Help your child learn that all-or-nothing thinking gets in the way of making changes and can lead to a pattern of restriction and overindulgence that not only doesn't feel good but reinforces negative eating and activity patterns. Remember, too, that when you let your child in on meal planning, food shopping and preparation, and planning family activities, she will learn to make good decisions from your example.

In fact, setbacks are a normal part of making any type of change. The key is not to get dejected. Instead, you and your child need to rethink what may have gone wrong and how you can minimize the risk of it happening again.

The first step in this process is to acknowledge that a setback has occurred or is still underway. Has your child stopped playing outdoors?

Is she spending more time in front of the television? Has the entire family started eating at fast-food restaurants more often than usual?

Once you give some thought to what might be going awry, the best corrections for your course may become rather obvious. Even so, you'd be surprised at how often parents and children know that something isn't going right but forget to take the time to evaluate what's really happening. That's why it might be helpful to write down what your child is eating and what her activity level is. The mere act of putting this information down on paper can help you identify specific problem areas and when and why they might be taking place.

Are the setbacks occurring when Grandma comes for a visit, for example? Does she bring some sweets with her that aren't ordinarily available in your home? Did your child go out for pizza or fast food 3 times last week, even though the family has been trying to stick to a once-a-week limit? Did you stop at the supermarket on the way home from work twice in recent days and buy some soda for the entire family? Does the setback follow periods of abstinence or withholding foods?

No matter what the problems are, they're now in the past. Rather than becoming frustrated or perhaps even scolding your child or other family members for these inevitable detours, acknowledge the fact that none of us are perfect. Stay optimistic. Turn your attention to health-promoting strategies. If your child is old enough, let her participate in this process of figuring out what went wrong and how you can prevent it from happening again.

If Grandma always brings a bag of candy whenever she visits, can you talk with her and suggest that she give her grandchildren nonfood gifts from now on? If you've backtracked from your commitment to cut back on trips to the local fried-chicken take-out restaurant, can you immediately do an about-face and return to healthier eating?

Once you reverse course and begin making positive changes, don't let down your guard and just assume that things will move forward without any further problems. Although some people think that they can make changes and then forget about them, you can't count on a smooth road ahead. You need to remain vigilant. Keep monitoring your child and family's progress in the weeks and months ahead. Make sure the family doesn't fall back into old habits that could undermine all the positive efforts to date.

Taking Action: Conquering Obstacles

Has your child experienced a lapse in his or her progress toward better health? If a setback does take place, use the following questions to help both of you understand and overcome the obstacles that may have tripped your child up. Remember, when trying to work through a setback, it's important to partner with your child's pediatrician.

What's Currently Happening?

- What setback has occurred in your child's life that has interfered with his or her weight-loss efforts? Did it happen just once or repeatedly? Is it still going on?
- Why do you think this backsliding has occurred? Is there an event, a person, or a behavior that has contributed to the problem?

What Changes Need to Be Made and How Will You Make Them?

- Think about a specific time in which a setback has occurred and where you and your child would like to make a change.
- Are there obstacles that you and your child need to deal with effectively to ensure success in preventing this setback from recurring in the future?
- What specific steps can you and your child take to make this change and minimize the risk of future setbacks?
- Who can support you and your child in making these changes?

Sneaking Food

It can happen at almost any time. While you're talking on the phone, when you're taking a shower, when you're out running errands— without your knowledge and perhaps without you ever finding out, your child may start sneaking food. When she's older, she may indulge at friends' homes, or when she has money, she may purchase her own snacks.

Why is your child behaving this way? After all, she may truly want to lose weight, so why is she sneaking food behind your back? There are many possible explanations. Your child could be feeling anxiety over issues with friends, and she might find food soothing and comforting. She could be bored or tired. Maybe she is reacting to an overly restricted diet she just tried. Or she may be sad or lonely. In many cases, she might interpret these emotions as hunger, and she'll raid the cupboard when no one's looking.

In most families, this sneaking of food doesn't go undetected for long. You might notice a few dirty dishes in her bedroom. Maybe there will be food items noticeably missing from the refrigerator. Perhaps you'll find candy wrappers in her wastebasket.

In cases like these, what should you do?

First, don't panic or overreact. Raise the issue with your child. Without being accusatory and becoming angry or threatening to punish her, tell your child that you've noticed that she sometimes eats in her room when she thinks no one is looking. Explain that you're aware of her behavior. Point out that it's counterproductive to her weight-loss goals. Then agree to help your child work on the problem.

Some parents find it helpful to establish a rule that their children have to ask them (or their spouses) for food. Rather than simply telling your child, "Don't sneak!" encourage her to ask for food when she wants it.

Explain that you'll help her make good nutritional decisions about what and when to eat. You can move her in the direction of sneaking less often and making better food choices when she does eat.

For example, you might say, "What kinds of foods have you been sneaking?"

Your child might respond, "I'm eating chips late at night."

You could follow up by asking, "Where do you get them?"

"I buy them from the vending machine at school."

"Well, when you feel like eating, can you make healthier decisions than reaching for chips? Next time you want some food, ask me. We'll choose foods together that can keep your weight-loss efforts moving in the right direction."

Once your child begins to ask you for food, reward her for doing so (although obviously don't reward her with food!). For a young child, give her a sticker or star each time she asks you for something to eat, or read her an extra bedtime story. She also can accumulate points for a low-cost toy or school supplies. For an older child, perhaps she can build up points for a ticket to the movies on Saturday afternoon or a day at the skating rink or zoo. Creating special time with your child when you do something fun together can help provide positive energy to make these healthy changes.

Your Child's Hunger

See if the following scenarios sound familiar:

- Your child sits down for dinner but only nibbles at her meal, eating very little of it. Then, 30 minutes after leaving the table, she comes into the kitchen, saying she's starving. Before you can utter a word, she starts eating something from the refrigerator or cupboard, and then returns again and again, grazing for food well into the night.
- Your child eats 3 highly structured, healthy meals a day that you carefully prepare, but then all those conscientious efforts toward good nutrition fall apart during her snacking, which at times seems as though it can turn into an all-day event.

For school-aged kids and adolescents, the biggest and most dangerous times for snacking are after school and after dinner. Typically, children will come home from school, and perhaps they're wound up, stressed out, or simply bored, so they reach for a pacifier in the form of food.

If your child seems to be overly reliant on snacking, look at what's going on. As a general guideline, children should consume 2 snacks a day, if needed—preferably healthy foods, such as fruits and vegetables. Of course, if the decision-making is left in their hands, many would opt for other types of snacks, like potato chips, cookies, candy, French fries, or a slice of pizza or two. If it's high in fat and rich in calories, it seems to draw them like a magnet. How about steering your child toward snacks such as

- Carrots or celery sticks
- A cup of melon or strawberries
- A cup of light microwave popcorn
- An apple
- A cup of vegetable soup

You can add to this list of healthy snacks. These are the kinds of foods that will help your child end of the cycle of unhealthy eating.

At the same time, recommit yourself to making sure your child eats 3 well-balanced meals a day; that should help quench her appetite for anything more than 2 modest and healthy snacks. If she's snacking out of boredom or anxiety, one of your challenges is to help her deal with the emotions and life situations that are steering her toward food. Encourage your child to take part in this decision-making. Ask her, "What can you do besides eat when you think you're hungry?" It sounds like a silly question, but some children will give it some thought and then say, "Well, I can go outside," "I can play with my toys," or "I can read a book." Those options are a lot healthier than feeding their hunger, particularly when it is being triggered by feelings or situations and not by the need for nutrition.

You may be surprised that your child can give you some alternatives to eating, or you may need to help her think of other things to do if she is stuck. Some ideas might be

- Walk the dog.
- Run through the sprinklers.
- Play a game of badminton.
- Kick a soccer ball.
- Paint a picture.
- Go in-line skating or ice-skating.
- Dance.
- Plant a flower in the garden.
- Fly a kite.
- Join you for a walk through the mall.

Teasing and Bullying

Some children with obesity have to deal with more than just losing their excess weight. They are also teased at school and even at home, often unmercifully, because of their weight. Over time, this taunting can take an emotional toll on any child, particularly if she loses friends and self-esteem. Some children eventually dread going to school at all. In fact, research shows that children who are bullied are more likely to skip going to class; some even drop out of school altogether.

In many cases, this taunting escalates with time. As it intensifies, children may become terrified, even fearing for their physical safety. For parents, it can be heartbreaking to watch.

So how should you and your child respond to this bullying?

- Tell an adult.
- Stay in a group.
- As much as she possibly can, she should not react to the taunting. If the school bully sees her becoming anxious or even start to cry, the teasing is likely to get worse. Encourage your child to maintain her composure, turn around, and walk away.
- Let your child's teacher know about the harassment being directed at your child. The teacher may be able to intervene to put an end to it. If the teasing continues, ask the school principal or your child's school counselor to get involved. Your child may be embarrassed to have you talk to the principal, but you can't afford to let her be mistreated any further. In fact, many schools now have anti-bullying policies. It is generally better to let the teacher and principal handle the situation, rather than contacting the bully or the bully's parents yourself.
- Encourage your child to try bonding more closely with the friends that she does have at school. If she hangs out with a group on the playground or in the lunchroom, she is less likely to be singled out for mistreatment.

- Add an activity outside of school that your child can participate in, during which she can develop a different peer group that may be less inclined to tease. Sign her up for a karate class or the scouts.
- Spend time with your child and treat her as an important person. Help maintain your child's self-esteem by demonstrating respect and acceptance and conveying the message, "I believe in you."

When you're evaluating the teasing to which your child is subjected, don't overlook what may be going on in your own home. Sadly, some children with obesity are teased by their own siblings. Even some parents direct negative comments at their child often, with statements like, "I'm telling you what to do—why aren't you doing it? You're just lazy." If this is happening in your home, you need to put a stop to it. Have a family discussion about it, and set some sensible ground rules for relating to one another in a more positive way. Chapters 11 and 12 delve more into the types of bullying and how to stay vigilant for any signs of bullying that may lead to a change in your child's eating or exercise habits.

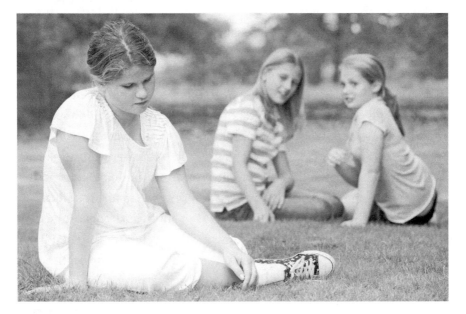

Child Care and School Issues

Because children spend so many hours a day in school or child care settings, one of your biggest parenting challenges is to stay up-to-date on what's going on there, including how it affects your child's health and well-being.

Of course, you should talk with your child daily about what's happening at school academically and socially. Who are her friends? Who does she eat lunch with? Where and what does she eat in the school cafeteria and from vending machines? Does she share food with friends, perhaps exchanging the lunch you've prepared with a friend's lunch?

In a growing number of schools, children can use a school debit card to buy lunches and snacks, with parents adding monetary value to the card every week or month. If your child uses one of these cards, how closely are you keeping track of how she's spending the money? If those funds are disappearing too quickly, your child may be overeating and perhaps making poor nutritional choices. With regularity, you need to ask her, "What did you buy with the debit card today?" If you're not pleased with the answer, you may need to switch strategies. For example, begin giving your child lunch money every morning so she can't overspend on items that she'd be better off not eating.

As we pointed out earlier in the book, you need to use the same hands-on approach if your child attends a child care center. Do you know what she's eating there? How much physical activity is she getting?

If you have concerns about your child's nutrition at the child care facility, find some time to talk with the child care teachers and inform them of your efforts to help your child maintain a healthy weight. Together, you should be able to work to make sure your child is eating healthy and getting a good amount of exercise. Some child care facilities even offer to send daily updates on what a child ate, what activities she participated in, and how she behaved.

Turn back to chapters 2 and 3 and review the suggestions made there for healthy eating and activity levels at school and child care. Remember to monitor what your child is eating. Even if you're having successes at home in improving her nutrition and activity level, the school environment can weaken those efforts if things are out of sync there.

When Time Becomes an Issue

Have you ever thought, "I know my child should be physically active, but there just aren't enough hours in the day! She's so busy with homework, art class, and after-school clubs that she just doesn't have time to get outdoors and run around." Or, "We made the decision to cut down on how often we eat out, but we're always so pressed for time. By the time I leave work and pick up the kids at child care, there's just no time to cook. Our goal of once-a-week restaurant dining ends up being 3 or 4 times a week."

Refrains like these are common among today's parents. If you plan ahead, there are solutions to just about every problem as your child works at managing her weight. For example, it might be true that time is limited for meal preparation on weeknights, but you can simplify things and do some advance planning on the weekends. As you read in Chapter 2, dinners don't have to be elaborate. They can be as simple as a sandwich, bowl of soup, piece of fruit, and glass of milk. It's easier to do the right thing than you might think.

How about the sixth grader who complains that she can't play outside for even 15 minutes because "I have too much homework"? You need to sit down with her and plan in advance for those days when it seems impossible to find even 15 minutes for physical activity. Create a schedule to fit in the most important (and healthy) tasks and activities that should be part of her after-school hours. It may be that while she does have plenty of homework, she might spend part of her homework time talking on the phone with a friend or texting her. It may be easier than you think to find those extra 15 minutes, particularly when physical activity is a family priority.

Also, have a plan B ready when things don't unfold the way you thought they would. Even if you arrange your child's schedule carefully, have a fallback strategy when unforeseen circumstances arise. At the last minute, maybe your child's math teacher changes the midterm examination from Wednesday to Tuesday, and suddenly your child will be studying well into the evening. Perhaps she has an orthodontist appointment that takes longer than you thought and, unexpectedly, there's much less after-school time than you had anticipated. In cases like these, your plan B might include some indoor activity for your child after dark (maybe the family can exercise together to a workout video), and dinner might be a frozen entrée that you had prepared over the weekend and placed in the freezer. Rather than letting events overwhelm you and your child, think ahead about how you'll handle the unexpected.

Keep in mind that there's a difference between being busy and being active. A lot of today's children are very busy with after-school activities, including tutoring and music lessons. Being busy, however, doesn't necessarily translate into being physically active, which is something children with obesity (and all children, for that matter) need. Kids must have balance in their lives, and exercise should be part of it. Activity needs to become a priority.

Vacations, Holidays, and Other Family Gatherings

Many children (as well as adults) tend to gain weight during holidays and vacations. On a weeklong trip to the beach, for example, families often let their nutrition and activity routines take a back seat to the events of the day. That's why it's helpful to think ahead and do some preparation before a vacation. Can the entire family agree to continue your healthy eating during your trip? Can you schedule some physical activity into your vacation, whether it's walking through the amusement park or swimming in the hotel pool? When you're on a trip, you shouldn't take a vacation from proper eating and exercise.

During holidays and other special occasions, don't lose sight of what your child is eating. Christmas and Hanukkah celebrations often last for much of December, with plenty of candy and cakes offering one temptation after another. In fact, for many families, the preoccupation with food extends from Thanksgiving through New Year's Day. No wonder you need to approach this time of year with extra care.

So how should you deal with the holidays? You certainly don't want to deprive your child of the celebrations. All of us, children and adults alike, need these kinds of celebrations in our lives. But celebrate the day, not the entire month! Your child can enjoy the holiday, departing from her nutritional plan for just a day, and then go back to her plan for healthy eating.

The same is true for birthday parties, other religious holidays, and Halloween. If your child is invited to a friend's birthday party, she can certainly have some ice cream and cake. But remind her to take only one helping of the treat. On Easter Sunday, for example, she can have a little candy, but fill up most of her Easter basket with inexpensive toys, and don't make Easter a 2-week celebration overflowing with sugar-laden goodies. On Halloween, let your child trick-or-treat but then suggest that she sell the candy to you for a negotiated amount. She'll get a few dollars, and you can dispose of the candy. Most children think that's a pretty good deal—besides, if the candy were to stay in the house instead, you just know someone would eat it! The key is to incorporate these occasions as parts of the family routine along with the family's day-to-day nutrition and activity patterns.

Now, what about other types of family gatherings? In some cultures, when extended families get together, it can turn into an absolute food feast, lasting from breakfast until the last light goes out after dark. Of course, extended families are important, but does your child need to have huge helpings of food whenever you go over to her favorite uncle's house? In fact, it's important to think moderation when you're at relatives' homes. Family members—grandparents, aunts, and uncles—can have an enormous effect on your child's health. Invite them to support her in her journey toward better health. Let them know that you'd like them to become part of your child's health team.

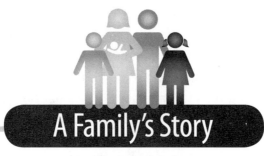

A Family's Story

Bullied at School

Jean, Bob, Jerry, and Melissa were enjoying their new healthy routine. Jerry even thought about joining the neighborhood baseball team. He had been practicing throwing and catching with his Dad and was starting to get comfortable hitting the ball on a regular basis. At recess one day, Jerry told his friends he was thinking of trying out. One of his friends, Harry, said, "You'll never make it. You are too big and slow." Jerry came home that day and told Jean he had changed his mind about trying out for the team. When he was getting ready for bed, Bob asked him what happened to change his mind and Jerry explained what Harry had said. Bob said that he could understand how hurtful Harry's comments were and that he was sorry Jerry had been teased. He reminded Jerry that it wasn't his fault Harry had said those mean things to him and that he had seen Jerry improve his swing enough to be a big help to the team. Jerry asked what to do, and Bob said that if Harry said anything to Jerry again, Jerry should just say he plans to try out for the team and then walk away. Bob asked Jerry to tell him if he was teased again and that he would talk with the teacher about what happened. Jerry ended up trying out and made the team.

Key Points to Remember

1 → Setbacks should be viewed as minor stumbling blocks and not a reason to abandon all efforts for healthy change.

2 → Monitor your child's progress and make certain she doesn't fall back into old habits with regularity.

3 → If your child is sneaking food, establish a rule that she has to ask you or your spouse for food so you can help her decide on a healthy snack.

4 → Children often snack not because they're hungry but because they're bored, anxious, or tired.

5 → When it doesn't seem as if there are enough hours in the day, plan in advance and set priorities so you can fit what's most important into your family's schedule.

6 → During holidays, your child should celebrate with the family and not feel denied. Even so, limits need to be placed on the amount of sweets that are available.

Chapter 7
Starting Early to Address the Risks of Obesity

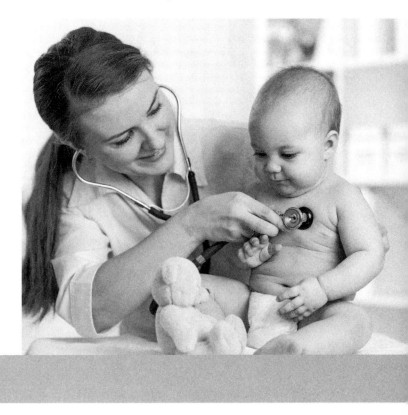

In this chapter and those that follow, we'll concentrate on specific developmental periods in your child's life and examine the issues most relevant to these times of life that may contribute to your child's risk of gaining weight. We will begin to look at the early risks that may lead to obesity and focus on the importance of your decision to breastfeed and the risks of obesity that come into play early on. Remember that it is always a good time to focus on improving your child's nutrition and activity, so if you have a child who has come into your life through adoption or foster care, you can start right where you are to make healthy nutrition and activity choices for your new arrival.

Good nutrition starts in the womb and during pregnancy. As a mother, your goal should be to get the best possible, most complete prenatal care, including paying attention to what you should be eating, your activity, and your weight gain.

The Early Risks of Obesity

It's vital to be aware of any obesity risk that could start even before your baby is born. If you, your spouse, or other close relatives have obesity, talk with your pediatrician about your baby's risk for developing a weight problem and how you can reduce that risk.

There are many factors that contribute to the risk of obesity for a child that begin in pregnancy. Some of the risk factors are important to know about even if you can't change them because they help you be extra-focused on a healthy lifestyle right from the start.

- Obesity in parents and other family members
- Obesity in mother even before pregnancy

Some factors that happen because of health problems can signal increased risk of obesity and need special attention from your health care professional.

- Excess maternal weight gain during pregnancy
- Diabetes or gestational diabetes in the mother
- Maternal smoking and secondhand smoke exposure
- Intrauterine growth retardation (babies born small for their age)
- Maternal antibiotic exposure in second or third trimester

You can address these factors before your baby is born by helping your family and home environment get in shape for a healthy lifestyle.

Optimizing Your Own Nutrition

With the guidance of your obstetrician, you need to eat a healthy diet that is right for you and your baby to thrive. If you have an overweight problem yourself or have been a constant dieter who latches onto one fad diet after another, your pregnancy is a time to set aside those diets and eat more healthfully, for your health and your baby's.

Your obstetrician will advise you to eat sensible, well-balanced meals that include extra calories, protein, minerals, and other nutrients to keep your baby growing well in the uterus. These nutrients will make their way to your growing baby, so be thoughtful about what you choose to put on your plate, making sure you consume a variety of healthy foods and beverages.

If your obstetrician recommends prenatal vitamin tablets, take them as suggested, but don't self-prescribe any other supplements until you discuss them with your doctor. You should also stay away from all medications, including over-the-counter pills, except those specifically recommended by your obstetrician. Many mothers have questions about taking certain medications (for example, cold or allergy medications) during pregnancy. This is normal; your obstetrician can answer these questions for you during prenatal visits.

The Decision to Breastfeed

The American Academy of Pediatrics (AAP) strongly recommends exclusive breastfeeding for about the first 6 months of age, which is about the age at which you'll start to add solid foods to his diet (see Where the American Academy of Pediatrics Stands box later in this chapter), and continued breastfeeding to age 12 months or longer as mutually desired by mother and infant. Mothers shouldn't feel guilty if they cannot breastfeed or if they decide to feed their baby formula. Formula can provide an adequate balance of fat, protein, and sugar that your baby requires.

There are many good reasons to breastfeed. Breastfeeding and breast milk

- Provide all the nutritional requirements that your newborn needs in the initial months after birth to grow and develop normally.
- Give your baby antibodies to help protect him against germs like bacteria and viruses, including those that cause ear infections, diarrhea, vomiting, urinary tract infections, pneumonia, and even bacterial meningitis. Breastfed babies also have a lower incidence of diabetes, asthma, and other chronic diseases and improved neurodevelopmental outcomes. Breastfeeding offers protection against sudden infant death syndrome.
- Allow mother and baby to bond emotionally during feeding in a special way. Breastfeeding encourages skin-to-skin contact between mother and baby, as well as time for cuddling with and comforting your baby.

- Are economical and, most mothers believe, more convenient—
they require no preparation (such as heating up a bottle) before
each feeding.
- Are the recommended feeding for preterm babies (babies born
3 or more weeks before their due date).
- Are healthy for mothers as well, significantly reducing their risk
for breast and ovarian cancer, cardiovascular disease, and
rheumatoid arthritis.

Breastfeeding is also important for obesity prevention.

- Breastfed babies who are breastfed for at least 6 months are less likely
to be overweight.
- The longer the duration of breastfeeding, the more reduction in the
risk of obesity. According to an article in the *Archives of Disease in
Childhood,* studies show that breastfeeding reduces the rate of childhood obesity. No, it won't eliminate your child's chances of becoming
overweight, but it does appear to have a definite effect on lowering
the risk.
- In a study published in the AAP journal *Pediatrics,* the rate of being
overweight was highest among children who were never breastfed
or were breastfed for less than 1 month, and there is a 15% to 30%
reduction in adolescent and adult obesity rates if any breastfeeding
occurred in infancy compared with no breastfeeding at all.

Although 80% of mothers expect to breastfeed, only 22% are
exclusively breastfeeding at 6 months. Critical periods for stopping
breastfeeding are

- Transition home from hospital
- Six to 8 weeks after birth
- Transition back to work
- Between 6 and 8 months due to self-weaning and/or introduction
of solids

These are times when the pediatrician, a lactation consultant, or peer breastfeeding support can help mothers stay the course and continue breastfeeding.

There are some medical conditions, medications, tests, and procedures for which breastfeeding is contraindicated (shouldn't happen). When deciding to breastfeed, it is best to check with your doctor about any medications you are taking or plan to take and any medical conditions that you may have.

In your initial meeting or two with your baby's pediatrician, talk with the doctor about how breastfeeding is going for you and your baby. Remember, there are no unimportant questions; the goal is to help you and your baby get the most out of breastfeeding. For more information about breastfeeding, check out HealthyChildren.org.

WHERE THE AMERICAN ACADEMY OF PEDIATRICS STANDS

In its 2012 policy statement about breastfeeding, the American Academy of Pediatrics confirmed its strong advocacy of exclusively breastfeeding babies for about the first 6 months after birth and supported continued breastfeeding for the entire first year after birth and beyond, as long as that is desired by mother and baby.

The policy statement also recommends having your pediatrician (or another experienced health care professional) evaluate your newborn when he is 2 or 3 to 5 days old (within 48–72 hours after discharge from the hospital), and again at 2 to 3 weeks of age, to be certain that he is feeding and growing typically. The checkup right after discharge is most important to make sure that your breastfeeding is coming along without any issues.

If you choose to start with formula feeding right after birth, it can be very difficult to switch to breastfeeding further down the road.

Your pediatrician may be able to recommend a lactation consultant or a class in breastfeeding to help you get started in breastfeeding. Lactation consultants are often nurses or dietitians with special training in teaching the fundamentals of breastfeeding and managing breastfeeding problems. Some of these consultants will come to your home after your baby is born if you're having difficulties. They will work with your pediatrician to help you successfully breastfeed your baby.

Physical Activity Starts in the Womb

Despite all the changes that are taking place in your body during pregnancy, this is no time to abandon your own efforts to stay physically active. Most women can exercise throughout their pregnancies, and it is important that mothers who are pregnant follow the advice of their obstetricians on the types of physical activity that are most appropriate for them. You might decide to take regular walks through your neighborhood, swim at the YMCA or in your backyard pool, or play golf. In general, most mild to moderate forms of exercise are healthy for you and your developing baby.

If you have certain pregnancy-related or preexisting health conditions, be sure to talk with your doctor before exercising.

The Home Environment

You and your family have spent months getting ready, painting and purchasing baby furniture, diapers, clothes, and toys, and now the big moment has finally arrived. But there is another environment that will have a big effect on your newborn as he grows, and that is your home and family environment. Healthy food in the pantry and refrigerator and the nutrition and activity spaces and places that promote physical activity and reduction of screen time, as well as the healthy lifestyle routines of the family, are all parts of a healthy home and family environment.

Think of your home environment as providing you, the parent or caregiver, with the tools you need to help your new baby have a healthy life.

If you have space in your home for movement, play, and tummy time, and have some balls and active games and toys, your baby has more opportunity to grow up moving and enjoying being active.

The nutrition environment you have at home has a strong influence on what your baby will eat once he starts solid foods. Pregnancy is a great time to evaluate the food in the house and make sure that healthy food is the easy choice for all family members. Here are a few tips.

- Make sure most food in the pantry and refrigerator is healthy food.
- If there are snacks and high-calorie foods, limit the amount and put them on the back shelf.
- Start transitioning to water and milk for the family instead of sugary drinks.
- Brush up on cooking skills to provide healthy meals and even homemade baby food.
- Schedule meals and snacks to develop healthy eating routines that limit grazing.

SELECTING A PEDIATRICIAN

Choosing a pediatrician is an important decision that you should make before your baby is born. Once your newborn arrives, it will be comforting to know that you have a pediatrician available who can care for your baby from birth, give him his very first examination, and answer all your questions.

New parents sometimes interview several pediatricians before making their choice. These interviews can usually be arranged during the last few months of your pregnancy. If you need the names of a few pediatricians, you can ask your obstetrician and check the American Academy of Pediatrics HealthyChildren.org Web site under "Find a Pediatrician." You can also ask friends and family members with children about the pediatricians they use and whether they're happy with their choice. You want to select a pediatrician who you feel you can talk to.

During your interviews with the pediatrician, ask questions like

- ► "How soon after birth will you see my baby for his first examination?"
- ► "At what intervals do you recommend seeing newborns for healthy baby visits?"
- ► "Are you willing to respond to questions by telephone, text, or e-mail?"
- ► "When you're unavailable, what pediatrician will I be able to reach instead?"
- ► "What procedures do you advise in case of an emergency?"
- ► "What are the fees for the health care services you provide, and do you accept the insurance my family has?"

Many additional topics discussed in this chapter and throughout the book can be raised during your interviews and subsequent visits to the pediatrician's office, including the benefits of breastfeeding and the prevention and management of obesity in children.

Key Points to Remember

1 The prenatal period is an important time to help ensure the good health of your baby.

2 Good nutrition starts in the womb. Be thoughtful about what you choose to eat.

3 Follow the advice of your physician to develop the right nutritional plan for you and your baby.

4 The AAP strongly recommends exclusive breastfeeding for about the first 6 months after your baby's birth, followed by continued breastfeeding as complementary foods are introduced, with continuation of breastfeeding for 1 year or longer as mutually desired by mother and infant.

5 Breastfeeding your baby may help to reduce his risk of becoming overweight.

6 Maintain an active lifestyle throughout your pregnancy with the guidance of your doctor.

Resources

American Academy of Pediatrics Section on Breastfeeding. Breastfeeding and the use of human milk. *Pediatrics*. 2012;129(3):e827–e841

Centers for Disease Control and Prevention. National Immunization Survey (NIS). https://www.cdc.gov/breastfeeding/data/nis_data/index.htm. Updated August 1, 2017. Accessed October 30, 2017

Centers for Disease Control and Prevention National Center for Chronic Disease Prevention and Health Promotion. Breastfeeding Report Card: United States/2014. https://www.cdc.gov/breastfeeding/pdf/2014breastfeedingreportcard.pdf. Published July 2014. Accessed October 30, 2017

Grummer-Strawn LM, Mei Z. Does breastfeeding protect against pediatric overweight? Analysis of longitudinal data from the Centers for Disease Control and Prevention Pediatric Nutrition Surveillance System. *Pediatrics*. 2004;113(2):e81–e86

Physical activity and exercise during pregnancy and the postpartum period. Committee Opinion No. 650. American College of Obstetricians and Gynecologists. *Obstet Gynecol*. 2015;126(6):e135–e142

Weng SF, Redsell SA, Swift JA, Yang M, Glazebrook CP. Systematic review and meta-analyses of risk factors for childhood overweight identifiable during infancy. *Arch Dis Child*. 2012;97(12):1019–1026

Yan J, Liu L, Zhu Y, Huang G, Wang PP. The association between breastfeeding and childhood obesity: a meta-analysis. *BMC Public Health*. 2014;14:1267

Chapter 8

The First Year

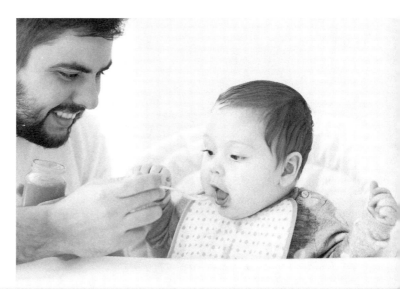

There are few life experiences more exciting than welcoming a new baby into the family. Even though it's such an exhilarating and enjoyable time for you and your partner, there are probably some moments when you simply feel overwhelmed. You might ask yourself questions like, "Am I doing everything right to get my baby off to a good start?" "Am I giving her all the nourishment she needs?" "What else should I be doing to make sure she stays on the path toward good health?"

Particularly if you, as parents, struggle with weight problems or have an older child who's overweight or has obesity, you might already be focused on how to prevent your new baby from developing a weight problem in childhood. Keep in mind, however, that your primary concern in this first year of your baby's life is not her weight, it's her overall health.

When your baby is born, her birth weight is influenced by a number of factors. Was she a full-term baby or born prematurely? Were there any complications during your pregnancy (for example, if mom's blood pressure was high while pregnant, the baby might be a little small)? Did mom consume a well-balanced diet during the 9-month pregnancy, or was her own nourishment deficient? Did you get regular prenatal care?

Now that your baby is born and is probably occupying many or most of your waking hours, your attention should be on her good health. Of course, during this first year after birth, you'll notice the normal baby fat that all babies have. Most babies appear a little chubby. Don't be too concerned. Trust your pediatrician to monitor your baby on a growth chart and let you know if she is growing normally. Ask to see your baby's growth chart, including weight for length chart, which is an index of your baby's nutritional status.

How Often and How Much Should Your Baby Eat?

It's important that you are attentive to clues or signals from your baby that indicate she's hungry. These are called *hunger cues*. When she wants to eat, she may become more alert, put her hands or fingers on or in her mouth, make sucking motions, stick out her tongue, smack her lips, kick or squirm, or begin *rooting* (moving her jaw and mouth or head in search of your breast). If she begins crying, this is usually a late signal that she wants to eat.

In most cases, she'll consume about 90% of the available breast milk during the first 10 minutes of feeding on each breast. Then she might move away from the breast or simply doze off. Among the many advantages of breastfeeding is that it tends to be cued or on-demand feeding, meaning that, in a sense, your baby will take charge of her own feedings. When you hold your baby to feed her a bottle, watch for cues that she is full, instead of using the clock as a guide. You might notice her becoming distracted while drinking from the bottle, or she might start fidgeting or turn her head from the nipple. She may close her mouth tightly. As your baby gets a little older and her eye-to-hand coordination gets better, she might try to knock the bottle or spoon out of your grip.

On the other hand, if your baby finishes a bottle and starts smacking her lips or begins to cry, she probably wants more. On average, by the end of the first month, she should be taking in at least 4 ounces of formula per feeding. At 6 months of age, she'll be consuming 6 to 8 ounces per feeding.

How Do You Know When Your Baby Is Full?

Whether breastfeeding or formula feeding, most parents worry about whether their baby is getting enough to eat. Because babies suck not only for hunger but also for comfort, this can be hard to know at first. Your baby should appear satisfied for a couple of hours after each feeding if she's consuming adequate amounts of food. Even when babies no longer act hungry, some parents worry about whether all their nutritional needs are being met. This is where your baby's pediatrician can help at her first well check at 2 to 5 days. Your pediatrician will measure her height, weight, and head circumference to make sure her growth is on target. This is also a time when you can talk with your pediatrician about your baby's feeding and any other concerns you have.

Table 8-1 shows that there are many ways babies can "tell" you that they are hungry and that crying or not going to sleep may have nothing to do with feeding (see A Crying Baby: What Does It Mean? section later in this chapter). We often don't think about how a baby looks, sounds, and behaves when she is full. Knowing the signs of fullness (called *satiety*) is another way of understanding your baby. You are like a detective, looking for clues about how your baby feels; you listen, observe your baby's movements, and see what she is paying attention to. Use Table 8-1 to help you read your baby's signals.

Age	Hunger Cues	Satiety Cues
Birth–3 months	Opens and closes mouth Brings hands to face Flexes arms and legs Roots around on your chest Makes sucking noises and motions Sucks on lips, hands, fingers, toes, toys, or clothing	Spontaneously releases nipple without searching for it again Moves head away from nipple Closes lips when attempting nipple reinsertion Slows or decreases sucking Extends arms and legs Extends/relaxes fingers Pushes/arches away Falls asleep
4–7 months	Smiles, gazes at caregiver, or coos during feeding to indicate wanting more Moves head toward spoon Tries to swipe food toward mouth	Bites nipple. Blocks mouth with hands. Turns away. Cries or fusses if feeding persists. Increases attention to surroundings. Loses interest in feeding. Releases nipple and withdraws head. Changes posture. Hands become more active. Keeps mouth closed. Plays with utensil. Shakes head "no."
8–12 months	Reaches for spoon or food Points to food Gets excited when food is presented Expresses desire for specific food with words or sounds	Shakes head "no." Hands bottle back to parent. Spits. Eating slows down. Clenches mouth shut. Pushes food away.

Table 8-1. Reading Your Baby's Hunger and Fullness (Satiety) Cues

Adapted from Trahms CM, Pipes PL, eds. *Nutrition and Infancy in Childhood.* 6th ed. New York, NY: McGraw-Hill and WIC Learning Online; 1997. https://wicworks.fns.usda.gov/wicworks/WIC_Learning_Online/support/job_aids/cues.pdf. Updated October 2016. Accessed October 30, 2017.

The Pediatrician's Role

To make sure your baby is growing well, your pediatrician will measure your baby's length and weight and then plot these measurements on the grow curve (figures 8-1–8-4). A measurement called *weight for length* can tell you and your pediatrician if your baby's weight is growing faster than her height; if so, your pediatrician will monitor your baby's feeding and activity.

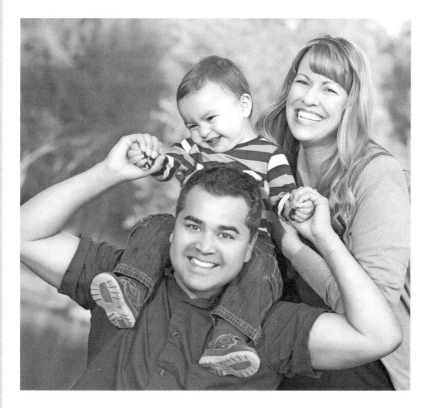

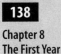

Figure 8-1. Head Circumference-for-Age and Weight-for-Length Percentiles, Boys, Birth to 24 Months

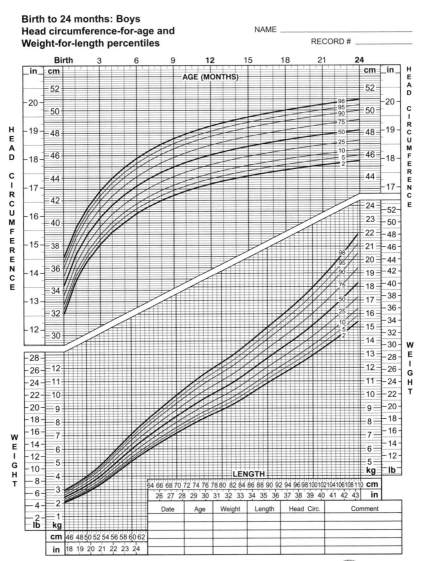

Birth to 24 months: Boys
Head circumference-for-age and
Weight-for-length percentiles

NAME _____

RECORD # _____

Published by the Centers for Disease Control and Prevention, November 1, 2009
SOURCE: WHO Child Growth Standards (http://www.who.int/childgrowth/en)

Figure 8-2. Head Circumference-for-Age and Weight-for-Length Percentiles, Girls, Birth to 24 Months

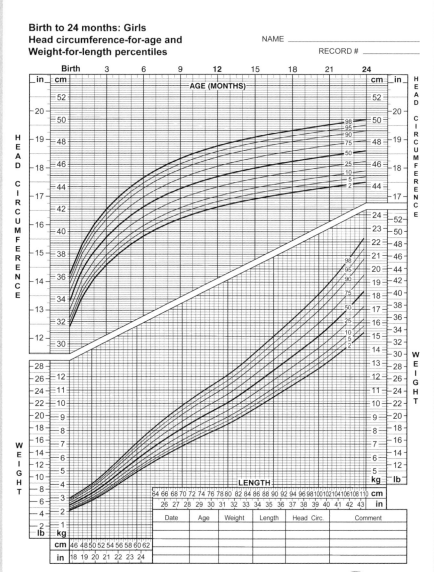

Published by the Centers for Disease Control and Prevention, November 1, 2009
SOURCE: WHO Child Growth Standards (http://www.who.int/childgrowth/en)

Figure 8-3. Length-for-Age and Weight-for-Age Percentiles, Boys, Birth to 24 Months

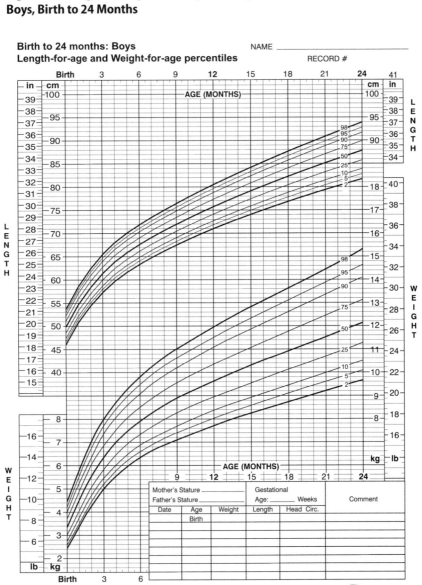

Birth to 24 months: Boys
Length-for-age and Weight-for-age percentiles

NAME

RECORD #

Published by the Centers for Disease Control and Prevention, November 1, 2009
SOURCE: WHO Child Growth Standards (http://www.who.int/childgrowth/en)

SAFER · HEALTHIER · PEOPLE™

Figure 8-4. Length-for-Age and Weight-for-Age Percentiles, Girls, Birth to 24 Months

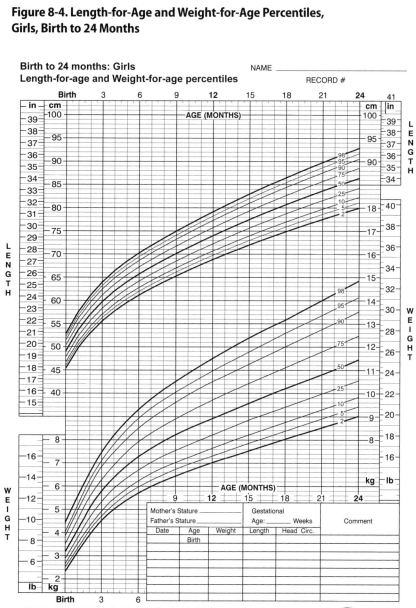

Published by the Centers for Disease Control and Prevention, November 1, 2009
SOURCE: WHO Child Growth Standards (http://www.who.int/childgrowth/en)

Getting Started With Solid Foods

Babies should start solid foods at about 6 months of age. You know when babies are mature enough to begin learning to eat from a spoon when they can

- Hold their necks steady and sit with support.
- Draw in their lower lips as a spoon is removed from their mouths.
- Keep food in their mouths and swallow it rather than push it back out on their chins.
- If you have any questions about your baby's readiness to start eating solid foods, consult with your pediatrician.

Introducing First Foods

According to the American Academy of Pediatrics (AAP) policy manual *Pediatric Nutrition,* 6 months is the starting point for gradual introduction of foods from all food groups, with new foods introduced one at a time every 3 to 5 days. For example, an infant cereal may be the first food, followed by meats, fruits, and vegetables. Remember, it is important for your baby to have healthy food from the start with no added sugar or salt.

A sample menu of what to feed your baby when she first eats solids is provided in the A Typical Menu for Your 8- to 12-Month-Old box.

Here are some additional recommendations to keep in mind.

- Introduce your baby to other solid foods gradually. By 7 to 8 months of age infants should be consuming fruits, vegetables, meats, dairy, and cereals.
- Start these new foods one at a time, at intervals of every 3 to 5 days. This approach will allow your infant to become used to the taste and texture of each new food. It can also help you identify any food sensitivities or allergies that may develop as each new food is started. Contact your infant's pediatrician if symptoms (for example, diarrhea, vomiting, rash) develop that seem to be related to particular foods.

A TYPICAL MENU FOR YOUR 8- TO 12-MONTH-OLD

Do you need some information and support in preparing a day's worth of meals for your infant? Your infant's pediatrician is the best source of this kind of guidance, but here is a sample menu of the daily food consumption for an 8- to 12-month-old. Use it to help you choose not only the types of foods for your infant but also the appropriate serving sizes.

1 cup = 8 ounces (240 mL)   4 ounces = 120 mL   6 ounces = 180 mL

Breakfast

¼–½ cup cereal or mashed egg

¼–½ cup fruit, diced (if your infant is self-feeding)

4–6 oz formula or breast milk

Snack

4–6 oz breast milk or formula or water

¼ cup diced cheese or cooked vegetables

Lunch

¼–½ cup yogurt or cottage cheese or meat

¼–½ cup yellow or orange vegetables

4–6 oz formula or breast milk

Snack

1 teething biscuit or cracker

¼ cup yogurt or diced (if child is self-feeding) fruit

Dinner

¼ cup diced poultry, meat, or tofu

¼–½ cup green vegetables

¼ cup noodles, pasta, rice, or potato

¼ cup fruit

4–6 oz formula or breast milk

Before Bedtime

6–8 oz formula or breast milk or water (If formula or breast milk, follow with water or brush teeth afterward.)

Adapted from American Academy of Pediatrics. *Caring for Your Baby and Young Child: Birth to Age 5.* Shelov SP, Altmann TR, eds. 6th ed. New York, NY: Bantam Books; 2014.

- In the beginning, feed your infant small serving sizes—even just 1 to 2 small spoonfuls to start.
- Within about 2 to 3 months after starting solid foods, your infant should be consuming a daily diet that includes not only breast milk or formula but also cereal, vegetables, fruits, and meats, divided among 3 meals.

When your infant is about 8 to 9 months old, give her *finger* foods or table foods that she can pick up and feed to herself. Make sure she's not putting anything into her mouth that's large enough to cause choking.

When Can I Give My Baby Finger Foods?

According to the AAP Web site for parents, HealthyChildren.org

- Once your baby can sit up and bring her hands or other objects to her mouth, you can give her finger foods to help her learn to feed herself.
- To prevent choking, make sure anything you give your baby is soft, easy to swallow, and cut into small pieces.
- Some examples include small pieces of banana, wafer-type cookies, or crackers; scrambled eggs; well-cooked pasta; well-cooked, finely chopped chicken; and well-cooked, cut-up potatoes or peas.
- Do not give small infants grapes, raw carrots, peanuts, raisins, nuts and seeds, popcorn, hot dogs, chunks of meat or cheese, hard or sticky candy, chunks of peanut butter, chunks of raw vegetables, or small or hard food pieces that can be easily aspirated. Cut foods in very small pieces no larger than one-half inch (see Chapter 9).
- Supervise all feedings (for example, do not let an older child feed an infant). You can find more information about choking hazards at HealthyChildren.org under choking prevention.
- Infants do best when they have routines for meals and snacks at predictable times.

How Active Is Your Baby?

You might not think of the first few weeks of your baby's life as being a time when she's very physically active. True, she's certainly not able to run through the park or throw a ball to another child at this age, but there are still many opportunities for her to begin to develop motor skills that she can build on for a very active childhood and adult life.

Tummy time is a way to help your baby enjoy being active and develop her motor skills. Find a space where you can put down a mat and sit or lay down next to her on the floor, and then enjoy!

LOW FAT? LOW CALORIES?

If you're concerned about your child's risk for obesity, you might be tempted to feed her only low-fat solid foods to help keep her weight at typical levels. Here's a very important recommendation to keep in mind: *Do not restrict your child's consumption of dietary fat and calories in the first 2 years after birth.* In other words, don't put a baby younger than 2 years on a diet or give her low-fat or skim milk unless recommended by her pediatrician.

Here's why: The early months and years of your child's life are critical for the normal development of her brain and body. Specifically, she'll need calories from dietary fat for her brain to grow and mature normally. As a general rule, your child should get about half her daily calories from fat up to the age of 2 years. After that, you can reduce those fat calories gradually; by 4 to 5 years, fat calories should provide about one-third of your child's daily calories. Many families transition from whole cow's milk to skim or fat-free milk by gradually changing from whole milk to 2% (reduced fat), and then to 1% (low fat), and then to skim milk. Some mothers even mix these together to make the changes imperceptible to their children.

Whether you've decided to breastfeed or formula feed your baby, either choice should provide your baby with all the fat she needs. However, when preparing formula, be sure to follow the label instructions carefully, adding the recommended amount of water. Formula is designed to provide about 20 calories per ounce, including the proper amount of fat to ensure optimal growth. If you weaken or dilute the formula by adding too much water, you can interfere with your baby's normal physical growth and brain development.

Here are a few tips for tummy time.

- Make sure your baby is awake and alert for tummy time.
- Place a mat on the floor with one or two safe toys appropriate for your baby's age.
- Lay down next to your baby and encourage her to look at the toys by describing the colors and shapes of the toys.
- Prop a baby book up so both of you can look at it and you can read to her or describe the pictures.
- Sing songs with her.

Have you noticed that your infant has started kicking by the time she is 2 months old? Even though this movement is mostly reflexive at this point, before long she'll be able to flex and straighten her legs whenever she wants to. By 3 months of age, your infant may be able to start kicking herself over from her front to her back. At about 3 to 4 months, when you hold her upright with her feet resting on the floor, she'll push down and straighten her legs as though she were standing on her own, and she'll probably discover that she can bend her knees and bounce.

Beginning at about 5 months of age, your infant will be able to raise her head while lying on her stomach and then push up on her arms to lift her chest off the floor or bed. Rocking on her tummy, she may kick her legs and move her arms as though she were swimming. Before long, your infant will be rolling over at will. She will begin to sit up at about 6 months and then, at about 8 months, she'll be able to sit without support and catch herself with her arms and hands if she starts to topple over. She'll also pick up and move objects from one hand to the other.

In the last few months before her first birthday, your infant may seem like she's in constant motion. She'll grab her feet and try putting them in her mouth. She may fidget and kick throughout every diaper change. Between 7 and 10 months of age, she'll begin experimenting with and then mastering the art of crawling. At 9 months, she can pull herself to a stand. Right around the time of her first birthday, she'll take her first steps (it may happen a little earlier or a little later from one child to the next, all within a typical range).

As your baby develops, take advantage of every opportunity to help stimulate her mind and body. From the earliest weeks after birth, walk around the house while holding your baby and interact with her by saying aloud the names of the objects that the two of you encounter. Before long, she'll want to reach out, touch them, and try to say their names. Also, talk to your baby whenever you're with her. Whether you're changing her diaper, bathing her, or driving with her in the car, keep the conversation going. Babies love the sound of their parents' voices. See how she responds and how she communicates with sounds by moving her arms and legs.

Here are some other activities that you and your baby can do together.

- Read out loud to your baby.
- Play some music and gently dance with her in your arms.
- For tummy time, sit and play with her on the floor. She will love interacting with you.
- Try teaching her peekaboo and pat-a-cake (they can be stimulating for your baby and will help her develop motor skills).
- Hug her frequently and provide her with loving physical contact.
- Hold your baby as often as you can.
- Go for a walk in the stroller. It's a good way to expose your child to the world around her, and it's great exercise for you.

As your baby continues to grow and develop, her level of activity will increase. Make sure she has safe and soft toys to play with. They should be small enough so she can pick them up but large enough so she can't put them in her mouth. The AAP recommends that families avoid digital media use (except video chatting) with children younger than 18 to 24 months.

For children aged 18 to 24 months, if you want to introduce digital media, choose high-quality programming and use media together with your child. Avoid solo media use at this age. Babies learn from watching and listening to you. Interaction with parents is the best way to help them learn and develop. Also, parents should note

- A television in the bedroom can interfere with getting to sleep and increase screen time, so keep the bedroom screen free.
- Start your child on a healthy bedtime routine; turn off the TV and read, talk, cuddle, and play.
- Screens at meals interfere with healthy eating and family time; make meals screen free.

Back to Sleep

Sometimes, it can seem like there is nothing more important than sleep. Babies need a lot of sleep, but as everyone knows, they don't sleep all at once, and your nights can feel like you are on a merry-go-round of waking up every 1 to 2 hours. Fortunately, babies get older and have more structured bedtimes and fewer interrupted sleep periods, and by about 6 months of age, they may be able to self-soothe themselves back to sleep when they wake up during the night.

Babies spend a lot of their time sleeping and need a safe sleep environment. The AAP has recommendations for safe sleep on HealthyChildren. org (see link in Recommendation for Infant Sleep Safety box). This is a must read for parents, from placing your baby on her back to sleep and crib safety to using a pacifier, bed sharing, and the effects of second-hand smoke.

RECOMMENDATION FOR INFANT SLEEP SAFETY

Until their first birthday, babies should sleep on their backs for all sleep times—for naps and at night.

For more information about safe sleep see the American Academy of Pediatrics video on safe sleep and the article "How to Keep Your Sleeping Baby Safe: AAP Policy Explained" on HealthyChildren.org (**https://www.healthychildren.org/ English/ages-stages/baby/sleep/Pages/A-Parents-Guide-to-Safe-Sleep.aspx**).

A Crying Baby: What Does It Mean?

When your baby cries, how do you react? Many parents instinctively think that she's hungry and needs to be fed. But there could be other reasons for her tears. Rather than immediately feeding your baby, take a moment to assess whether something else might be going on. Is she crying because she's uncomfortable, wet, or soiled? Is she sleepy? Is she having gas pains? Is she scared or irritated by noise and other stimuli that she finds too intense? Or is she ill (have you checked to see if she has a fever, for example)?

With time, you'll find yourself becoming much better at differentiating among your baby's cries. You'll know when she's very hungry or whether she just wants to be held or needs her diaper changed. Hunger cries tend to be short and low-pitched and rise and fall. A cry of distress or pain starts suddenly, is particularly loud, and tends to be a high-pitched shriek followed by a lengthy pause and then a flat wail.

No matter what the reason for your baby's tears, you should always respond to her needs. If you've just fed her, she's probably not hungry, and if nothing else seems to be awry, try letting her nurse some more or suck on a pacifier. Try rocking your baby or singing or talking to her. Gently stroke her head. Wrap her snugly in a receiving blanket, or walk with her in your arms or a stroller. The more time babies spend being held by their mothers, the less they cry. Remember, you cannot spoil a newborn.

Early Child Care and Education

Choosing a child care setting for your baby is an important decision. Whether you choose a child care center, family child care (this means an unrelated child care provider caring for your child in a family home), or a nanny, or have a family member help, you want the child care provider on your nutrition and activity team to provide the healthiest environment for your baby. Here are some tips to help you and your team.

- Find out the menu for meals, beverages, and snacks, and check to see if proper portion sizes and a variety of food groups are provided. You do not want your child to be given juice or other sweet beverages. If your child care is participating in the Child and Adult Care Food Program, it will be following the recommended food plans from the US Department of Agriculture Food and Nutrition Service (**https://www.fns.usda.gov/cacfp/meals-and-snacks**).
- Ask about tummy time, interaction with caregivers, and media use.
- If you are breastfeeding, make sure there is proper and safe storage of breast milk and a place for you to breastfeed when you are there.
- If your family is helping out, share what you have learned in this chapter with them so you can make a nutrition and activity plan for your baby that all family members can implement.

Key Points to Remember

The first year after birth is the perfect time to establish healthy feeding, sleeping, and activity routines.

Being responsive to your baby's hunger and satiety cues lays the groundwork for bonding and secure attachment and supports your infant's ability to manage hunger and fullness.

Interacting with your infant during tummy time, while reading or singing to her, or during her bath helps her develop her motor skills and makes these activities an enjoyable part of her routine.

Safety issues are important, and being aware of choking hazards of food and safe sleep are important for all caregivers.

Resources

American Academy of Pediatrics. *Caring for Your Baby and Young Child: Birth to Age 5.* Shelov SP, Altmann TR, eds. 6th ed. New York, NY: Bantam Books; 2014

American Academy of Pediatrics. Resources for families. Bright Futures Web site. https://brightfutures.aap.org/families/Pages/Resources-for-Families.aspx. Accessed October 30, 2017

American Academy of Pediatrics. Sleep. HealthyChildren.org Web site. https://www.healthychildren.org/English/ages-stages/baby/sleep/Pages/default.aspx. Accessed October 30, 2017

American Academy of Pediatrics. Starting solid foods. HealthyChildren.org Web site. https://www.healthychildren.org/English/ages-stages/baby/feeding-nutrition/Pages/Switching-To-Solid-Foods.aspx. Updated April 7, 2017. Accessed October 30, 2017

American Academy of Pediatrics Council on Communications and Media. Media and young minds. *Pediatrics.* 2016;138(5):e20162591

Centers for Disease Control and Prevention. Learn the signs. Act early. Developmental milestones. https://www.cdc.gov/ncbddd/actearly/milestones/index.html. Updated October 16, 2017. Accessed October 30, 2017

Daniels SR, Greer FR; American Academy of Pediatrics Committee on Nutrition. Lipid screening and cardiovascular health in childhood. *Pediatrics.* 2008;122(1):198–208

Chapter 9
The Toddler Years

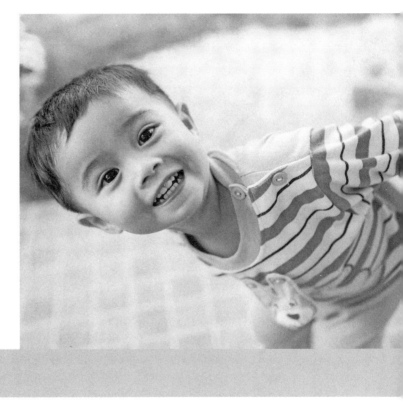

As your baby becomes a toddler, this can be a particularly pleasurable—and challenging—time for you as a parent. Although he's speaking in only 1- or 2-word sentences, he has enough language skills to communicate whether and when he's hungry and even verbally express his preferences about the foods he wants. At this stage in life, your toddler can feed himself with his hands, although he's also learning to use a spoon and drink from a cup. His food preferences may change frequently, and his appetite can increase or decrease from day to day, seemingly on a whim.

How Is Your Child Growing?

After his first birthday, your toddler's growth rate starts to slow, which is quite normal. Yes, his height and weight will increase steadily, but not as rapidly as it did in the first months after birth. On average, toddlers gain 3 to 5 pounds in their entire second year.

However, children of the same age can vary significantly in their sizes and rates of growth and still fall within the typical range. Despite these wide variations, you may be worried that your toddler is becoming overweight. You should express your concerns to your child's pediatrician, who can help you evaluate your child's individual growth. This is a time to aim for healthy nutrition and activity to support growth and development. This is best done in partnership with your pediatrician because there are risks when parents alter their children's diets in unhealthy ways.

This is also a good time to review how to read and interpret a growth chart, because the pattern of growth is what you and your pediatrician will be following to make sure your child maintains a healthy weight. You have already become familiar with the fact that an important part of the well-child check is measuring your child's height and weight and putting these results on a growth chart. Here is an example of how a toddler's growth can look over time.

Your son is 15 months old, weighs 23 pounds, and is 33 inches long. That means he is in the 50th percentile for weight and the 90th percentile for height, the same percentiles as when he was measured at 12 months old (Figure 9-1). This is because height and weight increase with age normally and tend to stay at the same percentiles. When he comes in for his checkup at age 18 months his weight is 28 pounds and his height is 35 inches. This puts his weight at the 90th percentile and his height at the 90th percentile (Figure 9-1). Clearly, something has changed.

To get a better idea of what his weight and height gain mean for his risk for obesity, your pediatrician will calculate his *weight for length,* which is plotted on another chart. At 15 months of age, his weight for length was in the 25th percentile, and at 18 months, his weight for length is in the 75th percentile. (For children younger than 2 years, there is no formal definition of obesity, but if your child's weight for length is above the 95th percentile, most pediatricians would consider that as being overweight.) When a child's weight for length starts crossing percentiles, like your son going from the 10th to the 75th percentile, you will need to discuss this change with your pediatrician.

Figure 9-1. Plotted Examples of Length-for-Age and Weight-for-Age Percentiles, Boys, Birth to 24 Months

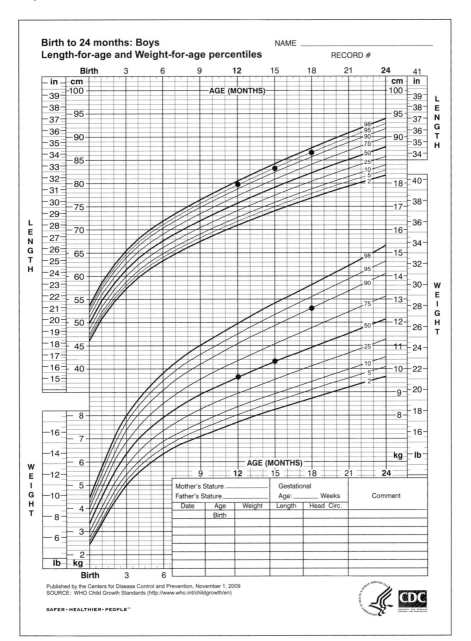

The Parent's Role

Although toddlers are beginning to develop food preferences, they also can be unpredictable about what they may want for a particular meal on a specific day. Their favorite food one day will end up being thrown on the floor the next. The food that they had spit out, day after day, will unexpectedly turn into the one they can't get enough of.

Picky eating is often the norm for toddlers. For weeks, they may eat 1 or 2 preferred foods—and nothing else. They may eat a big breakfast or lunch and then show no interest in eating much of anything else the rest of the day. Don't become exasperated with this kind of behavior. Just make healthy food choices available to your child in the appropriate portions, and acknowledge that his appetite or food preferences today may be quite different than yesterday's or tomorrow's. That's just the way toddlers are.

With time, your child's appetite and eating behaviors will reach an equilibrium. He'll find something he likes in a variety of healthy foods without much or any prompting from you. In the meantime, try working with picky eaters by giving them finger foods or table foods that they can feed to themselves. Just make sure these are healthy food choices, such as slices of banana or small pieces of toast. Also, avoid finger foods that could cause choking (see Preventing Choking box). Children don't fully develop the grinding motion involved in chewing until they're about 4 years old, so stick with foods that are small and easy to chew and avoid those that might be swallowed whole and get stuck in your toddler's windpipe. That means avoiding the foods listed in the Unsafe Foods for Toddlers box.

Even when your toddler is feeding himself, it's a good idea to sit with him while he eats. He's also old enough to join the rest of the family in eating at the dinner table. Use these family meals to model the healthy eating that you want your child to adopt for the rest of his life.

PREVENTING CHOKING

Your toddler's chewing and swallowing abilities aren't fully developed until 8 years of age. That means that he's more susceptible to choking and should be supervised while eating, whether at home or a child care setting. Here are some suggestions to reduce your toddler's risk of choking.

- Your toddler should be seated when eating. While sitting down, he's more likely to focus on the food in front of him and in his mouth.

- Don't allow your toddler to eat while in a moving car. As the car swerves or brakes, it could change the position of food in your toddler's mouth, leading to a choking episode.

- Round, firm foods, such as hot dogs, whole grapes, and apple chunks, are common choking dangers. Until your child is 4 years old, do not feed him any round, firm food unless it is chopped completely.

- Remind your toddler not to speak with food in his mouth. He should swallow food before talking.

UNSAFE FOOD FOR TODDLERS

Avoid the following foods, which could be swallowed whole and block the windpipe:

- ▸ Hot dogs (unless cut in quarters lengthwise before being sliced)
- ▸ Chunks of peanut butter (Peanut butter may be spread thinly on bread or a cracker, but never give chunks of peanut butter to a toddler.)
- ▸ Nuts—especially peanuts
- ▸ Raw cherries with pits
- ▸ Round, hard candies—including jelly beans
- ▸ Gum
- ▸ Whole grapes, cherry tomatoes (Cut them in quarters.)
- ▸ Marshmallows
- ▸ Raw carrots, celery, green beans
- ▸ Popcorn
- ▸ Seeds—such as processed pumpkin or sunflower seeds
- ▸ Large chunks of any food such as meat, potatoes, or raw vegetables or fruits

Adapted from American Academy of Pediatrics. Feeding & nutrition tips: your 2-year-old. HealthyChildren.org Web site. https://www.healthychildren.org/ English/ages-stages/toddler/nutrition/Pages/Feeding-and-Nutrition-Your-Two-Year-Old.aspx. Updated March 16, 2017. Accessed October 31, 2017.

The Pediatrician's Role

By now you know that your pediatrician won't rely solely on visual observation to determine whether your child's weight is at a healthy level. The most reliable guide is where your child's height, weight, and weight for length (for children younger than 2 years) fall on a standard growth chart. If the chart shows that your toddler is a little heavier than typical, your pediatrician can help you determine what actions are most appropriate at this age. As a general rule, however, you should never restrict calories in a toddler without the guidance of your pediatrician because you don't want to risk interfering with his normal growth and development. In evaluating his increase in weight, your pediatrician will ask about any signs or symptoms you've seen in your child and perform a physical examination to make sure he doesn't have any health problems that could be causing the weight gain.

The next thing is to see what could be causing him to gain weight more rapidly. Here is where the detective work begins. For most children, the proper health-promoting strategies are not complicated. They involve guidance that you've heard before.

- Optimize your child's nutrition.
- Make sure he gets plenty of physical activity and minimize screen time.
- Make sure he gets enough sleep.

An Action Step: Record Keeping

One of the most helpful things you can do as you try to unravel your child's weight gain is to keep a record of everything he eats and his physical activity, screen time habits, and sleep behavior.

This means that everyone caring for your child needs to keep track of what they are feeding him and what his sleep and activity schedule is like. This isn't as hard as it sounds because you are writing down the daily routines as you go. In general, 3 days of records, including the weekends, is enough to start to see patterns that are getting in the way of healthy eating, activity, and sleeping. You'll need to put in the amount and what kind of food your child ate or drank, wake-up and bedtime, length of nap time, and how much screen and playtime. Use Table 9-1 to record the information you've collected, or copy this template into a journal. If your child is with Grandma or in child care, ask if they can add to the record. You may be surprised at just how much is going on in your child's day!

Table 9-1. My Child's Daily Routine			
	Thursday	**Friday**	**Saturday**
Wake-up time Breakfast Screen time Snack Active play			
Lunch Nap Screen time Snack Active play			
Dinner Active play Screen time Bedtime			

Your Child's Healthy Eating

With your child's daily record in hand, you are now ready to see what is going well and what you may need to change to get him back to healthy eating. There is no question that since his very first feeding, you've probably paid plenty of attention to what your child eats, and now you are ready to take an even closer look. What should your toddler be eating? At 1 year of age, he should be consuming a wide variety of foods. As he moves through the second year after birth, he should be eating 3 meals daily, along with 1 to 2 snacks, prepared and served at regular times. You should also discourage grazing (this means your child has access to and grabs food all day long).

In planning and preparing food for your toddler, make sure he's getting a balance of fats, protein, carbohydrates, vitamins, and minerals that can promote growth by including a wide variety of foods each day.

- Vegetables and fruits
- Cereal grains, rice, potatoes, breads, pasta
- Meat, poultry, fish, eggs
- Dairy products, such as milk and cheese

One way to remember how to balance your child's meals and snacks is to refer to the picture of a well-balanced plate from the US Department of Agriculture ChooseMyPlate.gov Web site (**https://www.choosemyplate.gov**). This site has other helpful information for parents to plan healthy, well-balanced meals.

By choosing health-promoting foods, you can establish good nutrition habits in your child that will last for the rest of his life. However, one recent study found that about 65% to 70% of 1- to 2-year-olds ate dessert, ice cream, and/or candy once a day, and 30% to 50% drank sweetened beverages every day. By contrast, the same study indicated that fewer than 10% of these young children ate a dark-green vegetable each day; more often, their vegetable intake consisted of potatoes and French fries.

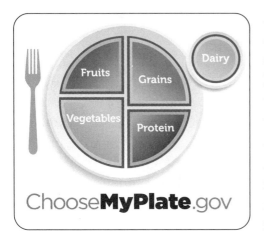

ChooseMyPlate.gov

Make sure that you and the other adults in the family agree on a healthy nutritional lifestyle for your toddler and the entire family, including one that puts a limit on sweets and sugar-sweetened beverages. An example of a healthy daily nutrition plan for a 2-year-old is in the Sample Daily Menu for a 2-Year-Old box.

For help in making good food choices, review the dietary recommendations in Chapter 2. On occasion, you'll run into unexpected disruptions that keep you from making a trip to the supermarket or spending time preparing meals in the kitchen. Everyone becomes sidetracked from time to time, so don't expect perfection. Even so, never lose sight of your objective, and stay headed in the right direction. Your goal should be to provide your child with a healthy, varied diet as regularly as possible, with choices from each food group. An occasional slipup—perhaps when, by necessity, the family is eating on the run—isn't going to undermine your toddler's good health.

What about portion sizes? They should be appropriate for your child's age. For a toddler, a serving size should be approximately one-fourth of the portion appropriate for an adult. A serving of vegetables for a toddler would be about 1 to 2 tablespoons. For meat, a serving might be about the size of his palm.

For your toddler, healthy snacking can be part of his daily diet. Here are examples of some appropriate snacks for this age group.

- Cut-up fresh fruits: bananas, apples, peaches, sliced pears, nectarines, plums (sliced and pitted), strawberries

---

SAMPLE DAILY MENU FOR A 2-YEAR-OLD

This menu shows a typical day of healthy eating for a 2-year-old who weighs about 27 pounds.

1 tablespoon = 3 teaspoons (15 mL)　　1 ounce = 30 mL

1 tablespoon = ½ ounce (15 mL)　　1 cup = 8 ounces (240 mL)

Breakfast	**Lunch**	**Snack**
½ cup nonfat or low-fat milk	½ cup low-fat or nonfat milk	½ cup nonfat or low-fat milk
½ cup iron-fortified cereal or ½ slice whole wheat toast	½ sandwich—1 slice whole wheat bread, 1 ounce cut-up meat, slice of cheese, veggie (avocado, lettuce, or tomato)	½ apple (sliced), ⅓ cup cut-up grapes, or ½ cut-up orange
⅓ cup cut-up fruit (for example, banana, cantaloupe, strawberries)		**Dinner**
	2–3 carrot sticks (cut up or cooked) or 2 tablespoons other dark-yellow or dark-green vegetable, cooked	½ cup nonfat or low-fat milk
1 egg		2 ounces cut-up meat
Snack		1/3 cup whole-grain pasta, rice, or potato
4 crackers with cheese or hummus or ½ cup cut-up fruit or berries	½ cup berries or 1 small (½ ounce) low-fat oatmeal cookie	2 tablespoons vegetable, cooked
½ cup water		

Adapted from American Academy of Pediatrics. *Caring for Your Baby and Young Child: Birth to Age 5.* Shelov SP, Altmann TR, eds. 6th ed. New York, NY: Bantam Books; 2014.

- Vegetables: peas (mashed for safety), potatoes (cooked and diced), steamed broccoli and cauliflower, green beans (well-cooked and diced), yams (cooked and diced)
- Meat and protein (cut up): fish, peanut butter (smooth, spread thin on a cracker or bread)
- Dairy foods: milk, yogurt (fresh or frozen), cheese (grated or diced), cottage cheese
- Breads and cereals: whole wheat bread, crackers, dry cereal, rice cakes

The Active Toddler

Physical activity is important for children of all ages. Of course, it may seem that your toddler gets all the exercise he needs as he's constantly on the move from sunup to sundown. He's crawling, walking, learning to run and jump, and kicking a ball or pulling toys behind him.

By 2 to 3 years of age, your child's physical activity will move to even more challenging levels. As his coordination keeps improving, he'll be able to walk up and down stairs. He'll run easily and start learning to pedal a tricycle. With his short attention span, he may be moving from one activity to the next, almost minute by minute, keeping you on the run just to keep up with him.

It is hard to overemphasize how important this active play is. Do not introduce the television (TV) to him until he is older; that way it isn't something attractive to him yet. The American Academy of Pediatrics (AAP) strongly believes that children up to 18 to 24 months of age should not be watching any screens (except video chatting with family); instead, they should be participating in supervised free play outdoors and indoors. Encourage them to play with siblings or plan playdates with neighboring kids or friends. When planning family activities, make them as active as possible, such as a hike or walking to the park.

You can also promote physical activity by using the stroller sparingly. When you're out for a walk, don't automatically sit your toddler in the stroller for the entire trip. Let him get out and walk beside you if that's what he wants to do.

If your toddler attends child care, ask the teachers how active he is there. Also, speak with the teachers about the meal plans and figure out ways to make sure your toddler is eating healthy amounts at designated and appropriate mealtimes. If snacks are given, ensure they follow your child's nutrition plan. Check to make sure the TV is not used often (if at all).

Action Step: Assessing Your Child's Healthy Living Environment

Ask yourself: *What are the things that are helping or getting in the way of my child's healthy weight?*

As a parent with a toddler in the house, one of your most important jobs is to understand what is happening to contribute to your child having a healthy weight or hindering him. Factors in your family, neighborhood, or community can play a role in how easy or hard it is to help your toddler who is gaining too much weight for his height.

In Figure 9-2, review all the factors that can play a role in weight gain. Circle each factor that you can identify that is affecting your child.

Remember, if you circle "Sugary drinks," consider this as something you can work on reducing or eliminating. Figure 9-2 is a useful tool to help you visually see the pros and cons present in your child's living environment.

Action Step: Set Routines

As parents, none of us would put our toddler in charge of picking out what we buy at the store, arranging our meals, or setting our bedtime. But, somehow, our children's wants work their way into our routines. Think of a time you were at the store and your toddler went immediately to the shelf and pulled off a toy. Did they calmly put it back after you said you weren't going to get it, or did you end up with a crying, inconsolable child? What about mealtimes; have you found yourself drifting toward chicken nuggets and fries because every other food gets a "no"? You can work your way out of this fix and into more healthy family routines, and here are a few tips on how.

Routines are important and help children feel calm and secure because they know what to expect. You may be having difficulty getting into healthy routines such as

- Mealtime behavior
- Bedtime

Figure 9-2. The Toddler Universe

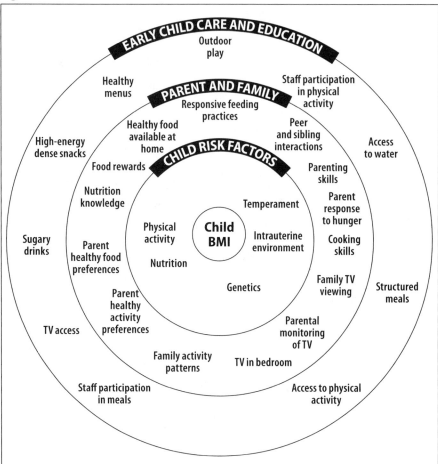

Source: Sandra G. Hassink, MD, MS, FAAP

- Grocery shopping
- Limiting TV time
- Snacking between meals (more than typical)

Here are some tips that may help for each situation.

SUGAR BABY

Studies have shown that any intake of sugar-sweetened beverages (soda, flavored milk, fruit drinks) in children aged 1 to 3 years is associated with an increased risk of obesity. Dessert, candy, and sweets, as well as sugary cereals, also contribute to an excess sugar intake in a toddler's diet. According to the American Heart Association, children younger than 2 years should avoid consuming any added sugars because they need nutrient-rich diets and are developing their taste preferences.

Here are some tips to reduce and eliminate added sugars from your toddler's diet.

- ▸ **"Sugar-proof" your kitchen and pantry.** Just like you made your house safe for your baby, you can make your house nutritionally safe by not having sugary drinks, sodas, candy, and sugary cereals at home.

- ▸ **Watch out for advertisements.** Toddlers recognize their favorite characters advertising sugary foods and will spot them on the boxes at the supermarket instantly.

- ▸ **Make fruits and vegetables a routine.** Build in variety and color and take advantage of nature's sweets. Make them easily accessible.

- ▸ **Be a good role model.** Have family members or other visitors not bring sweets or eat them around your child. Toddlers want to follow what others do.

- ▸ **Involve the family.** Grandparents love to give their grandkids sweets, candy, or soda. Sit down and talk about your desire and need to offer your child healthy foods and the powerful influence grandparents can be. The whole family can be good role models for the little ones. Remember, the most precious treat is time spent together.

Mealtime Behavior

- ■ Eating together as a family is very important. You are your child's first and most important role model for healthy eating and you can set, encourage, and continue this positive routine through adolescence. If your toddler is not eating with you every night, try to increase family meals by 1 extra time per week.

- ■ Sit your toddler in a high chair, put a cloth under the chair to make cleanup easy, and include your toddler in the family conversation.

- Have meals at the same or similar times every day as much as possible. It is easier for children (and adults) to manage their hunger if they know when the meal is coming.
- Pick specific times for snacks, make them healthy, and have your toddler sit in his high chair to eat them.
- Serve your toddler (and the rest of the family) healthy food in the right portions. It is easier to eat the right amount when the serving bowls are not right on the table.
- Let your toddler decide how much and what to eat, choosing from the healthy food you put on his plate. Don't worry if he doesn't eat everything; he is learning when he is full.
- Include one or two foods in the meal that you know your toddler will eat, so you don't have to worry about him refusing everything.
- Put one new food in your meal and his meal. If your toddler sees the whole family enjoying it, he may be more willing to try it too.

Bedtime

Bedtime routines are comforting and help settle in for the night. Think about what you want to include in your routine.

- Reading a book can be a special time with your child and increase his vocabulary and reading skills, and when you read to your child you are getting him ready to learn at school.
- A bath is calming and can be a good time for some quiet downtime with your child.
- Singing quietly or talking about your day can be wonderful additions to a bedtime routine.
- Set a time for bed and start your routine with enough time to make sure your toddler is ready to sleep.

Grocery Shopping

- Have your child point out colors or shapes of food items.
- Help your toddler name the fruits and vegetables.
- Let your child place a nonbreakable food item into the cart.
- Try not to go shopping when you or your toddler is hungry.

Limiting TV Time

- Just like meals and bedtime, *you* should pick the times you want you and your toddler to watch TV.
- Turn off the TV during meals and snacks. Background TV interferes with your child's interaction with you and may create a habit for your child in thinking the TV should be on during these times.
- Watch TV with your toddler, so you can interact with him during the show and distract him during the commercials.
- Do not put a TV in your child's bedroom
- Make most time TV-free. Ensure that toys are accessible and stimulating for your child. When you can, get down on the floor and play with him.
- For AAP guidelines on media use for young children, see Table 9-2.

Snacking Between Meals

It is hard to hear your toddler say that he is hungry and not automatically reach for the easiest and most convenient snack, like chips or cookies, but many things besides needing food for energy can trigger the feeling of hunger. Some of them are

- Boredom
- A TV commercial for food
- Seeing another family member eating or drinking
- Being tired
- Being thirsty
- Associating a situation with food, such as playdates or grand-parent visits
- Seeing food on the counter (Fruit is OK.)

When your child says he is hungry, stop and think. Ask yourself the following questions:

- When was his last meal or snack? If he missed a snack or is due for a meal, you can serve that meal or snack now.
- Is your child bored? Have a list in your head of simple distractions he likes, such as coloring, reading a book, or playing a game.

(continued on page 174)

Table 9-2. American Academy of Pediatrics Media Use Guidelines for Young Children

Age	Description	Media Use Guidelines
Younger than 2 y	Children younger than 2 learn and grow when they explore the physical world around them. Their minds learn best when they interact and play with parents, siblings, caregivers, and other children and adults.	For children younger than 2, • Media use should be very limited and only when an adult is standing by to co-view, talk, and teach. For example, video-chatting with family along with parents.
	Children younger than 2 have a hard time understanding what they see on screen media and how it relates to the world around them. However, children 15 to 18 months of age can learn from high-quality educational media, IF their parents play or view with them and reteach the lessons.	For children 18 to 24 months, if you want to introduce digital media, • Choose high-quality programming. • Use media together with your child. • Avoid solo media use.
2–5 y	At 2 years of age, many children can understand and learn words from live video-chatting. Young children can listen to or join a conversation with their parents. Children 3 to 5 years of age have more mature minds, so a well-designed educational program such as *Sesame Street* (in moderation) can help children learn social, language, and reading skills.	For children 2 to 5 years of age, • Limit screen use to no more than 1 hour per day. • Find other activities for your children to do that are healthy for their bodies and minds. • Choose media that is interactive, nonviolent, educational, and prosocial. • Co-view or co-play with your children.

Adapted from American Academy of Pediatrics. Healthy digital media use habits for babies, toddlers & preschoolers. HealthyChildren.org Web site. https://www.healthychildren.org/English/family-life/Media/Pages/Healthy-Digital-Media-Use-Habits-for-Babies-Toddlers-Preschoolers.aspx. Accessed October 31, 2017.

WHERE THE AMERICAN ACADEMY OF PEDIATRICS STANDS

▶ In the first 2 years after birth, your child's brain and body are going through very critical periods of growth and development. During this time, it is important for your child to have positive interactions with other people, including adults and children, and not sit idly in front of the TV.

▶ For that reason, the American Academy of Pediatrics currently recommends that families avoid digital media use (except video chatting) in children younger than 18 to 24 months. For children aged 18 to 24 months, if you want to introduce digital media, choose high-quality programming and use media together with your child. Avoid solo media use in this age group.

▶ For children 2 to 5 years of age, limit screen use to 1 hour per day of high-quality programming, co-view with your children, help children understand what they are seeing, and help them apply what they learn to the world around them.

▶ Avoid fast-paced programs (young children do not understand them as well), apps with lots of distracting content, and any violent content.

▶ Turn off TVs and other devices when not in use.

▶ Avoid using media as the only way to calm your child. Although there are intermittent times (eg, medical procedures, airplane flights) when media is useful as a soothing strategy, there is concern that using media as strategy to calm could lead to problems with limit setting or the inability of children to develop their own emotion regulation. Ask your child's pediatrician for help if needed.

▶ Monitor children's media content and what apps are used or downloaded. Test apps before children use them, play together, and ask children what they think about the app.

▶ Keep bedrooms, mealtimes, and parent–child playtimes screen free for children and parents. Parents can set a "do not disturb" option on their phones during these times.

▶ No screens 1 hour before bedtime, and remove devices from bedrooms before bed.

- If he is asking for something he just saw on TV, limit TV time and have him play a game or play with toys.
- If an older sibling or family member is eating between meals and snack time, get that person into the family meal and snack schedule.
- Think about whether your child is tired or thirsty. A nap or a glass of water may be just the thing.

HUNGER PAINS

Battling these types of challenges can be difficult for any parent. Here's an example of your child being hungry outside of a typical lunch hour while grocery shopping with you. Consider how you would handle this situation.

You are rushing out of the house to get some grocery shopping done in time to come home and make dinner. You've just picked Jeffrey, your 2-year-old, up from child care, and he's asking for a snack, which you forgot to pack because you were late getting home from work and in a hurry to get to the store.

You get to the store and the first thing he see is a box of cookies at the entrance to the market. He asks for the cookies and within a few seconds begins to cry that he is hungry and he wants them. He runs up to the display and grabs a box and tries to put them in your cart. You say "no," and he starts to scream.

Your choices are

- Keep saying "no" and put the cookies back.
- Leave the cart and the store and take him home.
- Apologize to everyone who is watching as he throws a tantrum and let it run its course until he is worn out.
- Buy the cookies.

Being in a rush is part of our daily lives, but no one wants to end up in this situation if it can be helped. What can you do to keep this from happening again?

- Have healthy snacks ready to go at home and put one in your car.
- Make sure he has his snack and a drink of water and explain what the shopping trip will look like before heading into the store. For example, try saying, "Jeffrey, we are shopping for food for dinner so I can get home and cook. You can help me by looking for the lettuce, OK?"
- Bringing a toy or comfort item from home may also keep him distracted enough from tempting items.

Life can be busy, but with a little planning ahead you can help reduce your stress and get everyone home in good shape.

Key Points to Remember

You are the most important role model for your child—what you eat, the home environment you create, and the routines you establish all set the stage for your child's healthy life.

Having a plan for responding to your child's behavior, whether he is a picky eater or is having tantrums, eases the way for you to make healthy changes for your family. Your child's pediatrician can help if you have questions about your child's behavior.

Busy toddlers are not necessarily active toddlers. Play is a toddler's exercise, building muscles and coordination. Scheduling time for safe free play is a priority in this age group.

Enlisting the aid of all who care for your child (for example, grandparents, child care, babysitters) in developing healthy routines sets the stage for a healthy childhood.

Resources

American Academy of Pediatrics. Choking hazards parents of young children should know about [video]. HealthyChildren.org Web site. https://www.healthychildren.org/English/safety-prevention/at-home/Pages/Choking-Hazards-Parents-of-Young-Children-Should-Know-About.aspx. Updated July 26, 2017. Accessed October 31, 2017

Blum RE, Wei EK, Rockett HR, et al. Validation of a food frequency questionnaire in Native American and Caucasian children 1 to 5 years of age. *Matern Child Health J.* 1999;3(3):167–172

Dattilo AM, Birch L, Krebs NF, Lake A, Taveras EM, Saavedra JM. Need for early interventions in the prevention of pediatric overweight: a review and upcoming directions. *J Obes.* 2012;2012:123023

Dwyer JT, Suitor CW, Hendricks K. FITS: new insights and lessons learned. *J Am Diet Assoc.* 2004;104(1 suppl 1):s5–s7

Fox MK, Pac S, Devaney B, Jankowski L. Feeding infants and toddlers study: what foods are infants and toddlers eating? *J Am Diet Assoc.* 2004;104(1 suppl 1):s22–s30

Harrington JW, Nguyen VQ, Paulson JF, Garland R, Pasquinelli L, Lewis D. Identifying the "tipping point" age for overweight pediatric patients. *Clin Pediatr (Phila).* 2010; 49(7):638–643

Ogden CL, Carroll MD, Kit BK, Flegal KM. Prevalence of childhood and adult obesity in the United States, 2011-2012. *JAMA.* 2014;311(8):806–814

Pan L, Li R, Park S, Galuska DA, Sherry B, Freedman DS. A longitudinal analysis of sugar-sweetened beverage intake in infancy and obesity at 6 years. *Pediatrics.* 2014;134(suppl 1):S29–S35

Stettler N, Kumanyika SK, Katz SH, Zemel BS, Stallings VA. Rapid weight gain during infancy and obesity in young adulthood in a cohort of African Americans. *Am J Clin Nutr.* 2003;77(6):1374–1378

Vos MB, Kaar JL, Welsh JA, et al. Added sugars and cardiovascular disease risk in children: a scientific statement from the American Heart Association. *Circulation.* 2017;135(19):e1017–e1034

Chapter 10

The Preschool Years

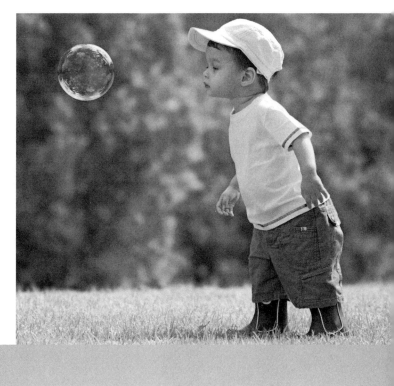

Your child's body has undergone significant changes since the day you brought her home from the hospital. By now, as she moves through her preschool years, your child's baby fat has been replaced by increases in muscle development, accompanied by a slimming of her arms and legs and a tapering of her upper body. Many children at this age still have a small potbelly or pear shape.

Some children of this age appear skinny, and their parents often worry that their children are undernourished or perhaps have illnesses that make them look thin. Then there's the other end of the spectrum, where parents worry about something quite different. Their children are heavier than their playmates. These kids may be eating larger meals and snacking more often than their peers. They might be watching more hours of television (TV) and spending fewer hours being physically active. This is a good time to take stock and begin to move your child and family to a healthier lifestyle.

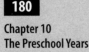

The Parent's Role

As you move your child and the rest of the family in the direction of healthier eating, you'll also find that preschoolers have already developed clear food preferences, but that these preferences may change from one day to the next. Kids might favor a particular food one day, perhaps even ask for seconds—and then refuse to eat the same food the following day. They may insist on eating a specific food for several days in a row, and then push it away on the days that follow. Don't make this kind of behavior a point of contention; it's quite normal in children at this age. Just be sure that your child is being given healthy choices at every meal. As a parent, your job is to provide your child with good nutritional options in the proper portions each day, and then let your child decide whether to eat some or all of it, depending on how hungry she is or her preferences on that particular day. Don't stop serving vegetables, for example, just because your child pushes them away during one or several meals. If you back away from preparing and giving her vegetables or anything else that might not be one of her favorites, you could eventually end up with a child who eats only peanut butter and French fries!

In choosing portion sizes for your child struggling with weight, start by giving appropriately sized servings; if she asks for more, try vegetables and fruits. If she persistently requests extra helpings, try slowing the pace of the meal down, offering a salad as a first course, or adding a protein to the previous meal or snack to decrease hunger. Younger children in your family should be served smaller portion sizes than older siblings and parents. Meals and snacks should be structured, meaning that you should provide your child with appropriate portions and choices at appropriate times that fall in line with the family meal schedule.

This type of structured eating helps children manage their hunger and reduces the likelihood of inappropriate snacking. On the other hand, if your child snacks or grazes all day long, she'll probably cherry-pick her favorite foods during regular meals, rather than eating the healthy foods you are serving. (For guidance on proper portion sizes, refer to Chapter 2, which provides examples of serving sizes for 4- to 6-year-olds.)

SAMPLE DAILY MENU FOR PRESCHOOLERS

This typical menu was designed for a 4-year-old weighing about 36 pounds.

1 teaspoon = ⅓ tablespoon (5 mL)   1 ounce = 30 mL

1 tablespoon = ½ ounce (15 mL)   1 cup = 8 ounces (240 mL)

Breakfast	**Lunch**	**Dinner**
½ cup nonfat or low-fat milk	½ cup nonfat or low-fat milk	½ cup nonfat or low-fat milk
½ cup whole-grain cereal	1 sandwich—2 slices whole wheat bread with 1–2 oz of meat and cheese, veggie, and dressing (if needed) or peanut butter and jelly	2 ounces meat, fish, or chicken
4–6 oz or ½ cup cantaloupe, strawberries, or banana		½ cup pasta, rice, or potato
		¼ cup vegetable
Snack	¼ cup dark-yellow or dark-green vegetable	*If your family would like to include margarine, butter, or salad dressing in any meal, choose low-fat or healthier versions, if possible, and only give 1 or 2 teaspoons to your child.*
½ cup nonfat or low-fat milk	**Snack**	
½ cup fruit such as melon, banana, or berries	1 teaspoon peanut butter with 1 slice whole wheat bread or 5 crackers or string cheese or cut-up fruit	
½ cup yogurt		

Adapted from American Academy of Pediatrics. *Caring for Your Baby and Young Child: Birth to Age 5*. Shelov SP, Altmann TR, eds. 6th ed. New York, NY: Bantam Books; 2014.

Remember, meals don't have to be elaborate to be nutritious and support a weight-control effort. You can prepare a healthy meal in minutes—a turkey sandwich, serving of peas or green beans, piece of fruit, and glass of milk. In fact, many young children prefer simple foods, so on days when you're pressed for time, there's no need to spend 45 minutes in the kitchen preparing dinner.

What your child drinks is important, and sugary beverages have excess calories, add risk for obesity and cavities, and don't provide any nutritional value. The American Academy of Pediatrics (AAP) recommends that, for children aged 4 to 6 years, fruit juice should be restricted to 4 to 6 ounces daily, and children should be encouraged to eat whole fruits instead of drinking fruit juice. This adds fiber and increases the feeling of fullness without the extra calories of juice.

When it comes to snacks, don't leave snack food out on the kitchen counter that your child and siblings can grab whenever they want. Limit snacks to 2 per day, and provide your kids with healthy choices. Instead of candy or chips, offer them fruit, a slice of low-fat cheese, finger sandwiches, or reduced-fat or natural peanut butter on crackers. Desserts like cake and ice cream are fine occasionally but not as a daily routine.

You should also work to cut down on your family's visits to fast-food restaurants. Unless you're very selective about what your child eats there, she can end up consuming more fat, sugar, salt, and calories than she does at home, sabotaging your efforts at promoting good nutrition and effective weight management.

PREVENTING CHOKING

Your child's chewing and swallowing abilities aren't fully developed until 8 years of age. That means that she's more susceptible to choking and should be supervised while eating, whether at home or a child care setting. Here are some suggestions to reduce your preschooler's risk of choking.

▶ Your child should be seated when eating. While sitting down, she's more likely to focus on the food in front of her and in her mouth.

▶ Don't allow your child to eat while in a moving car. As the car swerves or brakes, it could change the position of food in your child's mouth, leading to a choking episode.

▶ Round, firm foods, such as hot dogs, whole grapes, and apple chunks, are common choking dangers. Until your child is 4 years old, do not feed her any round, firm food unless it is chopped completely.

▶ Remind your child not to speak with food in her mouth. She should swallow food before talking.

When you go, make an effort to choose healthy options like fruit and milk rather than fries and soda. By limiting, the consumption of high-calorie foods and sweets, you'll not only ensure that your family is eating a more nutritious diet today, but you'll lay the groundwork for healthy eating habits that can last for the rest of your child's life.

Your child and the rest of the family should try to balance their eating on a daily basis. However, if your child or others in the family have a day when they've eaten too much or have had too little physical activity, take a step back and say to yourself, "This was today; tomorrow's a new day." Variations in eating patterns and activity are inevitable but don't need to derail your efforts to achieve a healthy lifestyle.

Calculating Body Mass Index

Although kids come in all different shapes and sizes, more children today measure at an unhealthy weight than in previous generations. Your child's pediatrician has been charting her height and weight since she was an infant, typically during every office visit in the first 2 years after birth and then about once a year thereafter. Your pediatrician also calculates your child's body mass index (BMI).

Body mass index is a number that is calculated by dividing your child's weight in kilograms (kg) by her height in meters squared (m^2) (or dividing her weight in pounds [lb] by height in inches squared [in^2] and multiplying by 703). After the BMI for your child is calculated it is plotted on a graph. Separate graphs are used for boys and girls (figures 10-1 and 10-2). The BMI graph shows where your child is in comparison to a population of children her age before the obesity epidemic started. From the graph, you can then use the symbols key to see if your child is underweight, a healthy weight, or overweight (Table 10-1).

Table 10-1. Body Mass Index Classification		
Category	**Symbol**	**Description**
Underweight	■	<5th percentile
Normal or healthy weight	★	5th percentile to <85th percentile
Overweight	▲	85th to <95th percentile
Obese	●	≥95th percentile

Figure 10-1. Body Mass Index, Boys, 2 to 20 Years of Age

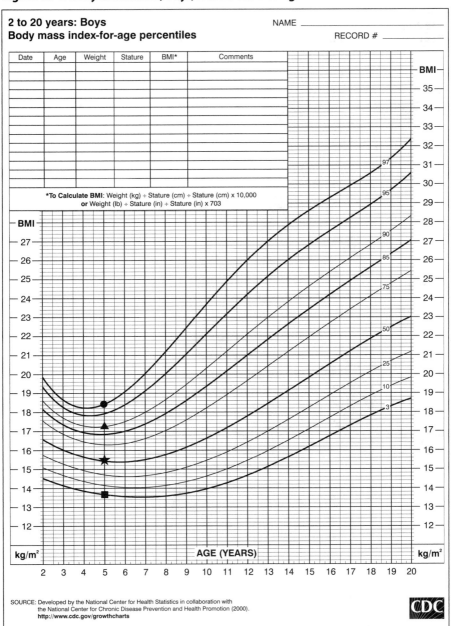

2 to 20 years: Boys
Body mass index-for-age percentiles

NAME _____

RECORD # _____

Date	Age	Weight	Stature	BMI*	Comments

*To Calculate BMI: Weight (kg) ÷ Stature (cm) ÷ Stature (cm) x 10,000
or Weight (lb) ÷ Stature (in) ÷ Stature (in) x 703

AGE (YEARS)

kg/m²   kg/m²

SOURCE: Developed by the National Center for Health Statistics in collaboration with
the National Center for Chronic Disease Prevention and Health Promotion (2000).
http://www.cdc.gov/growthcharts

CDC

Figure 10-2. Body Mass Index, Girls, 2 to 20 Years of Age

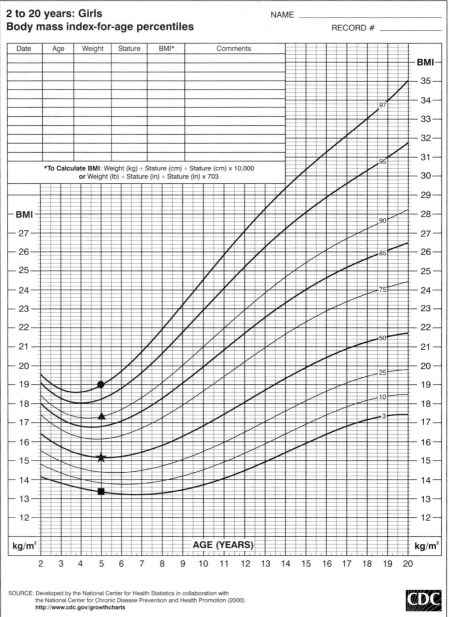

2 to 20 years: Girls
Body mass index-for-age percentiles

NAME _____

RECORD # _____

*To Calculate BMI: Weight (kg) ÷ Stature (cm) ÷ Stature (cm) x 10,000
or Weight (lb) ÷ Stature (in) ÷ Stature (in) x 703

SOURCE: Developed by the National Center for Health Statistics in collaboration with
the National Center for Chronic Disease Prevention and Health Promotion (2000).
http://www.cdc.gov/growthcharts

The Pediatrician's Role

The preschool years are a time when a growing number of children are first identified as having an elevated BMI. If your child has a BMI above the 85th percentile, your child's pediatrician will do 3 things.

Obtain a Growth History

Your pediatrician will look at your child's growth over time to see when her weight began to increase faster than her height and her BMI began increasing. This gives your doctor a picture of when there might have been a change in your child's lifestyle or health that resulted in increased weight gain (or decreased height growth). Knowing this time frame can often provide clues to help get your child back on track to a healthy weight.

Medical Evaluation

Your pediatrician will review a detailed history of your child's health to make sure that she doesn't have any rare health condition that could cause extra weight gain or health problems caused by her extra weight gain. Your doctor will also review her medications and ask about family history, focusing on any obesity-related chronic health conditions. Along with this, your pediatrician will perform a physical examination. Your pediatrician may also order specific laboratory tests as part of the medical evaluation.

Nutrition and Activity Assessment

Your pediatrician will ask specific questions about diet, physical activity, and lifestyle to get a picture of your child's daily eating and activity routines.

What's in Your Pantry?

If your preschool-aged child has obesity or is overweight, you'll probably need to make some adjustments in her diet. Rather than focusing primarily on cutting down on calories, for example, most of your attention should be placed on ensuring that she eats a variety of healthy foods each day. Make certain that she's eating balanced meals served in portions that are appropriate for her age. (Restricting calories carries potential risks in a growing child, so you should do so only under the supervision of your child's pediatrician.)

Your entire family should show their support and join the effort to reshape your household's nutrition. To help you make optimal food selections for your family, refer frequently to the information in Chapter 2 and the AAP book *Nutrition: What Every Parent Needs to Know,* keeping in mind that these are guides, and not prescriptions.

FOOD INSECURITY

Families may have times when providing enough food for their children is a struggle and they are experiencing food insecurity. Your child's pediatrician may already be asking your family 2 questions that lets your doctor know that your family may need help getting enough food. These questions are

1. Yes or no? Within the past 12 months, we worried whether our food would run out before we got money to buy more.

2. Yes or no? Within the past 12 months, the food we bought didn't last and we didn't have money to get more.

If the answer is "yes" to either or both questions, there is a good chance your family is experiencing *food insecurity.* In that case, your pediatrician can provide information to help make connections with federal food programs, like SNAP (Supplemental Nutrition Assistance Program) or WIC (Special Supplemental Nutrition Program for Women, Infants, and Children), or the federal summer feeding programs in your community, as well as community food pantries. Check with your pediatrician to get help with finding food resources. You can also call the US Department of Agriculture national hunger hotline for more information: 1-866-3-HUNGRY (866/348-6479) or 1-877-8-HAMBRE (877/842-6273).

Action Step: Pantry Planning

One of the best ways to make sure your family's food environment is healthy is to take an inventory of what is in your pantry. This can be done with the whole family. Using Table 10-2 as a template, write down how many of each types of food you find in your pantry, counting all the fruits, vegetables, low-fat dairy, lean protein, and whole grains. When you are finished, compare the numbers and see which food groups you have a lot of and in which areas you need more. This will be your guide for planning future meals and snacks.

| Table 10-2. Pantry Planner: Healthy Foods ||
Type	Amount
Fruits	
Vegetables	
Low-fat dairy	
Lean protein	
Whole grains	

| Table 10-3. Pantry Planner: Less Nutritional Foods ||
Type	Amount
Foods and drinks	
Sugary drinks	
Salty snack food	
Sugared cereal	
Candy and cookies	

Now calculate the other foods in your pantry and refrigerator (Table 10-3). These are the foods and beverages that are likely to lead to increased calorie consumption. They are foods with very low nutritional value for the energy they provide. You may want to eliminate or buy very little of these foods to make your house as healthy as possible.

Remember, only have the foods and beverages in the house that you want your child to eat; anything else is just temptation.

Managing Screen Time

Preschoolers are developing habits that will last a lifetime, so managing screen time and creating healthy activity time is laying down an important foundation for the rest of their lives.

Eating and Television

There is plenty of unconscious eating that can take place in front of the TV, with children snacking their way from one program to the next, so make it a rule that there is no eating in front of the TV and that the TV is off during mealtimes. This applies to tablets and phones as well. Your child should have her meals with other family members as often as possible so mealtimes can become a valuable time for family conversation and sharing the day's experiences.

Eating and Advertisements

There's another important downside to excessive TV watching. Hour after hour, your child will be exposed to a steady stream of TV advertising, much of it for high-sugar, high-fat foods, often linked to favorite cartoon characters. More often than not, impressionable preschoolers will tell their parents that they must have the particular type of cereal or sweet with the character's picture that they've seen on TV, making it even harder to keep kids traveling on the road to healthier eating. Studies have shown that children who watch a lot of TV have a greater likelihood of developing obesity, and the commercials targeted at children are one of the reasons why.

Screens and Activity Time

Children as young as 3 years who are inactive tend to keep this pattern of inactivity throughout their childhood into their adult years. Screen time is a big reason why more children are preferring indoor time to going outdoors and electronic games to more interactive indoor pursuits. Scheduling screen time has become a must, and making time for outdoor play or family activities needs to come first. Once your child gets into a screen time routine, she will take it for granted and you will have established a healthy activity and screen time routine that fits within your family's lifestyle. The AAP advises that your child's daily screen time limit should not exceed 1 to 2 hours of screen viewing, including time spent playing computer and video games. For help making a plan for managing screen time, refer to the AAP family media plan at **www.HealthyChildren.org/MediaUsePlan**.

Increasing Physical Activity

Your preschool-aged child may seem like she has an endless supply of energy, enough to keep her active for most of the day and night. Too often, that energy never gets used. Because some preschoolers may spend hours a day in front of the TV, their high energy levels go to waste, giving rise to an increased risk of developing obesity. Today's children are much less active in their day-to-day lives than their grandparents were. That kind of statistic is troubling and calls for parental intervention.

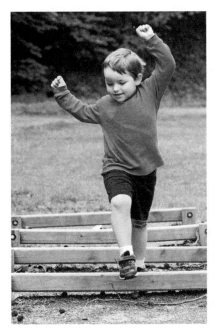

Keeping your child physically active is another effective way of combating obesity. During a child's preschool years, you should encourage free play as much as possible, which will help her develop motor skills and her imagination. At this age, improving coordination will make your child more agile and allow her to participate in games and activities with greater skill. Even more important than turning to highly structured activities, find safe and adult-supervised opportunities where your child has time for unstructured play, which is crucial to development. In a real sense, play is a child's work, and it is key to helping her grow physically as well as socially, emotionally, and intellectually.

Watch your child during these times of spontaneous play and you'll see how her motor skills are improving. Rather than darting aimlessly from one activity to another, she'll be much more interested in (and capable of) playing tag with other kids or riding her tricycle for long periods. She'll become adept at catching a bounced ball and throwing a ball overhand. She'll run, skip, hop, jump, and walk up and down stairs without holding onto the railing. She'll perform somersaults and climb on playground apparatuses. She'll also develop creativity and problem-solving abilities, learn to cooperate with playmates, and discover the world around her.

Provide your child with age-appropriate play equipment, from balls to plastic bats, to make exercise fun, but let her choose exactly what to play with at any given time. When you're planning family time, schedule physical activities whenever possible, whether going for a bike ride on the nearby bike path, kicking a soccer ball back and forth in the local park, or playing catch in the backyard. Remember, parents are important role models for physical activity.

Keep in mind that your preschooler's physical skills are developing far faster than her good judgment. Her playtime needs to be supervised, particularly to keep her from dangerous situations, like chasing a ball into the street.

CHILD CARE GUIDANCE

If your preschooler spends time in a child care setting, she should be physically active for much of that time. Safety must be the first priority. Does the child care facility provide safe outdoor and indoor play areas for your child and other kids? Is your child always supervised, not only during play periods but while eating? Is the food your child is being served there compatible with the nutritional goals you're trying to reach at home? (If not, ask for changes in lunch or snacks.) Are your child and others seated while eating or running around with food like raw carrots in their hands and mouths, increasing the risk of choking? If your child care sends home notes or pictures of what your child has done that day, this is a terrific way to get a glimpse into her eating and activity behaviors. If not, you could ask if this could become a possibility.

If your preschooler has obesity and is on a weight maintenance eating plan, make sure the child care providers know what dietary restrictions she has. They need to be partners in this effort toward normalizing your child's weight, and if they're feeding your child high-fat snacks, insist on some healthier alternatives.

What if Your Child Becomes Resistant?

When you're making changes in your family's lifestyle that may involve everything from what you put on the kitchen table to how often you allow the TV to be turned on, don't be surprised if your preschooler or other family members are annoyed (or worse) at times. If you're going to help your child manage her weight, you can expect some groaning and complaining and even some outbursts of anger. Other changes, like fewer trips to fast-food restaurants or more physical activities for the entire family, could elicit some grumbling and whining. If you're not careful, you might be tempted to give in to the anger and complaints by letting your child have her way, but this approach, although easier in the short term, will work against the long-term change your child needs to achieve a healthy lifestyle.

To reduce the likelihood that your child will react with anger, make sure that the changes you're making apply to your entire family. If you serve your child different foods than others at meals and snacks, she'll feel singled out and isolated. If everyone is eating a healthy dish of

fruit as a dessert, however, she's much more likely to accept it as
the new way of doing things.

When angry outbursts do occur, it's good to already have a plan in place
to deal with them effectively. Talk with the other adults in the home and
agree in advance on how you all will respond to these temper tantrums
about your family's lifestyle changes. Here are some suggestions.

- **Stay calm.** Don't react to your child's anger by becoming irritated
  yourself. That will only put you and your child on a collision course
  and escalate the difference of opinion rather than resolve it. A lot
  of parents take their child's outbursts personally and end up lashing
  out themselves, which is never helpful.
- **Give a time-out.** Perhaps have her sit in a chair for a few minutes
  and tell her, "When you can talk nicely, you can come back into the
  family room." Time-outs work if you're consistent and remain calm.
- **Stay the course.** Never lose sight of the fact that you're making these
  long-term changes for the health of your child and family, and explain
  that to your child. Say something like, "We all want to be healthy, and
  just like all of us buckle our seat belts to keep us safe in the car, we're
  going to eat a little differently, too, so we stay healthy." Don't give in to
  her insistence that she turn on the TV, and don't make deals. Avoid
  statements like, "OK, just this once I'll let you watch cartoons until
  dinnertime, but then you can't ask me to do it again tomorrow." If you
  hold your ground, your child will realize that all her complaining is a
  waste of energy, and these episodes are likely to decrease in frequency.
  It is important to be consistent and follow through with what you
  have said. If you don't, and you give in, you will reinforce your child's
  behavior to bug you until you give in again.

If you decide to reward your child for good behavior and willingness
to follow the new family rules, don't use food as a reward. Positive
attention, praise, or a hug are often all the reward she needs. Perhaps
give her a sticker or read an extra bedtime story. The best gift to give
your child is your time and doing something that is enjoyable.

What if Your Child Is "Always Hungry"?

We have all had the experience of wanting to eat when we know we have had enough. For example, the smell of baking cookies can make us want to grab a handful, or seeing a commercial for a fast-food meal can make us want to run to the nearest fast-food restaurant. We can all remember being stressed and reaching for the closest food, such as chips or ice cream. Random hunger pangs can come from a whole host of reasons and occur even if you have just eaten, and your child is no different.

As parents and family members, we are programed to offer food to a child who says she is hungry, and we do this almost without thinking. But if we stop a minute and think about what our child has eaten that day, when her last meal or snack occurred, and then ask ourselves whether she could be bored or tired, we can get to the bottom of her hunger. Here are some tips for handling those random hunger pangs.

- **Try hard to keep meals and snacks to a schedule.** It is much easier to ask a child to wait if she is hungry at 5:30 pm and dinner will be at 6:00 pm, than if dinner could be anywhere from 6:00 to 8:00 pm.
- If your child says she is hungry and you think she may be bored, **have a "things you can do" list** that you and your child create together and ask her to pick something from it. If she comes back again, keep working off the list.
- **Playing outside** is a great way to limit screen time and a cure for boredom. Activities such as playing catch, drawing on the sidewalk with chalk, and shooting baskets with a kid-sized basketball hoop are great substitutes for grazing.
- Hunger is often triggered by seeing food on the counter, especially snacks and sweets. **Try not to have food in the house you don't want your child to eat.** Put healthy fruit and snacks right up front on the shelves or in the fridge.

What Would You Do?

You have just picked your 4-year-old up from preschool after a stressful day at work. It's 5:30 pm and she runs to the car, gives you a hug, and says she is hungry and wants a snack. You let her know how glad you are to see her and that you are going right home to cook spaghetti, her favorite! She starts to whine and says she can't wait and doesn't like spaghetti and wants something else. You're tired, and you have taken her to the store before for a cookie and juice. You know she would be happy with this snack and calmer when you are trying to cook dinner.

You may feel that your only choices are

- Tough it out—reassure her that dinner will be ready soon and try to distract her.
- Tell her you will get her a snack as soon as you get home.
- Go to the store and try to find a healthy snack.
- Go to the store and buy the cookie and juice.
- Be firm that spaghetti is dinner tonight but that you can go home and both pick out a healthy snack for her.

Late afternoon, after work and preschool, can be one of the most stressful times of the day for you and your child. What can you do to keep this from happening again? Here are some tips.

- Find out what is on the menu for meals and snacks at your child's preschool and ask how much she is eating. This will help you get an idea if she is avoiding some foods or holding out for the snack food she wants when you pick her up.
- Plan easy family dinners on work nights; even a sandwich, salad, fruit, and milk will do. Choose meals that are quick to prepare to lessen the time your child has to wait for her meal.
- If you know dinner will be awhile, pack a healthy snack for your child when you pick her up to eat before you drive home.

- If you have time and can get outside for 15 minutes before going home, this may be the break she needs after a day in preschool.
- Have a coloring project or book for her to look at on the ride home.

Key Points to Remember

1 → Be calm and consistent. Remaining calm in the face of a tantrum and keeping to the healthy routines you have decided to follow will make moving you and your preschooler toward a healthier lifestyle a smoother journey.

2 → Getting other family members and caregivers on board with healthy eating and activity is important. Your preschooler depends on the adults in her life to make sure she stays healthy.

3 → Even though your preschooler is busy exerting her independence, you are still the captain of the ship and need to provide healthy food in the right-sized portions for meals and snacks.

4 → Planning for supervised free play is the best way to encourage physical activity in your preschooler. Free play helps to restore energy balance, improve motor skills, and foster imagination.

Resources

American Academy of Pediatrics Committee on Injury, Violence, and Poison Prevention. Prevention of choking among children. Pediatrics. 2010;125(3):601–607

American Academy of Pediatrics Council on Communications and Media. Media and young minds. Pediatrics. 2016;138(5):e20162591

American Academy of Pediatrics Council on Community Pediatrics and Committee on Nutrition. Promoting food security for all children. Pediatrics. 2015;136(5):e1431–e1438

American Academy of Pediatrics, Food Research and Action Center. *Addressing Food Insecurity: A Toolkit for Pediatricians.* http://www.frac.org/wp-content/uploads/frac-aap-toolkit.pdf. Published February 2017. Accessed October 31, 2017

Burdette HL, Whitaker RC. Resurrecting free play in young children: looking beyond fitness and fatness to attention, affiliation, and affect. *Arch Pediatr Adolesc Med.* 2005;159(1):46–50

Heyman MB, Abrams SA; American Academy of Pediatrics Section on Gastroenterology, Hepatology, and Nutrition and Committee on Nutrition. Fruit juice in infants, children, and adolescents: current recommendations. Pediatrics. 2017;139(6):e20170967

Chapter 11

The School-age Years

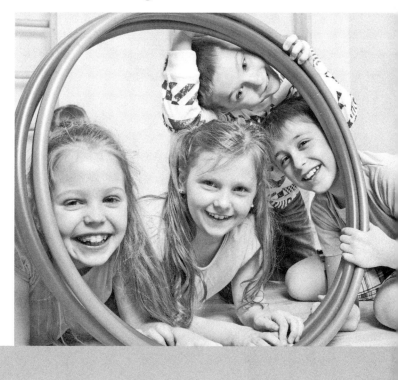

Every stage of your child's life presents challenges for you and your child, and this includes the school-age years. During this time in his life, your child will be adjusting to new educational and social settings, interacting with more children than ever before, and making many new friends. He'll also be developing new academic skills and increasing his knowledge of the world. All the while, he'll be relying on you for advice and guidance.

During these years from ages 6 through 12, children need good nutrition to keep growing normally. As they approach adolescence, most girls experience increases in their growth rate, on average, between the ages of 10 and 12 years, while boys will begin their greatest growth spurts about 2 years later. Some parents worry that throughout the school-age years, there seems to be no rhyme or reason to their children's appetite. One day, they may eat everything in sight, while on other days, they might turn into such a finicky eater that you'd expect their stomachs to be growling throughout the day.

Making Sense of Childhood Eating Behaviors

In most cases, unpredictable eating patterns even out, and as long as your child's pediatrician tells you that your child is growing normally and his weight, height, and body mass index (BMI) are on target, keep your focus on offering a variety of healthy foods, keeping him in an active routine, and ensuring he gets enough sleep.

Children in this age group, like the rest of us, may eat for a lot of reasons besides hunger. Even when they complain that they're starving, hunger may not be the reason why they want something to eat. They could be

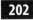

upset or tired and relying on food for comfort. For some children, eating may merely be a habit—for example, they're used to eating snack foods anytime they're watching television (TV) or playing video games. When your child says that he's hungry and it's not a regular mealtime or snack time, try to determine if food might be serving some other purpose, and then problem-solve. If your child seems to be bored, for example, help him find an activity that will keep him occupied doing something productive and steer him away from food. Distracting your child's hunger with a fun, physical activity is one way of achieving 2 goals.

If your child is struggling with his weight, both of you have some additional challenges. In many families, when children have been heavy since their preschool years, their parents expect—or at least hope—that this weight problem will finally resolve itself as young bodies grow and mature from the ages of 6 through 12 years. That often doesn't happen. Shortcomings in nutrition and inadequate physical activity that began early in life often continue throughout childhood, unless a conscious effort is made to change course. For example, even though there are many ways for your school-aged child to be physically active, the TV and video or phone games may be winning the battle for your child's time and attention. As a result, his weight might continue to climb.

At each visit to your pediatrician's office, the doctor calculates your child's BMI (see Introduction) and can tell you whether he's exceeding the normal range on standard growth charts. During the school-age years, children gain weight at a steady rate to match their growth; as they approach puberty, those increases in weight will accelerate. If your pediatrician has raised some red flags, cautioning you about your child's excessive weight gain, you need to take them seriously. Children who have obesity are much more likely to have obesity as adults, which will place them at risk for serious chronic disorders, such as heart disease and diabetes. However, with the support of your pediatrician, this is a time when you and your child can make changes that direct him along the proper path toward better health. As your pediatrician may tell you, these are very important years for helping your child adopt healthy eating and activity habits that can last a lifetime. These are also important years for your child to develop self-esteem and confidence, which can be damaged by weight-based bullying and teasing. Being bullied can affect your child's emotional health and lower his self-esteem, which, in turn, can lead to a cycle of inactivity and overeating. By taking steps like offering your child appropriate foods in the right amounts and encouraging him to be physically active every day, any weight concerns that exist now will become less of a problem as he gradually moves toward the typical/healthy range on your pediatrician's growth chart.

The Parent's Role

During these middle years of childhood, there are plenty of obstacles that can trip up your well-intentioned efforts at keeping your family eating right. Children spend most of their weekdays at school, and that is why they need the healthiest possible food served at school breakfast, at school lunch, after school, and at school events. As a parent, you need to know what kinds of meals and snacks are being offered during and after school. Many schools have Web sites on which they list the school menu. This is a good chance to check out what is offered and go over healthy choices with your child in advance. A healthy school lunch should look like the one found on ChooseMyPlate.gov (**https://www.choosemyplate.gov**).

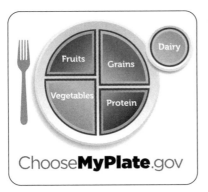

As a parent, you will be trying to find solutions for any stumbling blocks that arise. If the school cafeteria doesn't offer many healthy choices or your child cannot be convinced to purchase healthy options (and in many elementary and middle schools, only one lunch entrée is provided), there are several things you can do.

- Pack a healthy lunch for your child each day. You might prepare a turkey sandwich on multigrain or pita bread. A peanut butter and jelly sandwich is fine too. There are plenty of good selections, but stay away from pastrami, salami, and other high-fat lunch meats.

> ### CHOOSEMYPLATE GUIDE TO SCHOOL LUNCH FOR FAMILIES
>
> ▸ **Grains:** Whole grains give kids B vitamins, minerals, and fiber to help them feel fuller longer so they stay alert to concentrate at school.
>
> ▸ **Vegetables:** A variety of vegetables helps kids get the nutrients and fiber they need for good health.
>
> ▸ **Milk (low fat [1%] or fat free):** Children and teens need the calcium, protein, and vitamin D found in milk for strong bones, teeth, and muscles.
>
> ▸ **Fruits:** Every school lunch includes fruits as well as vegetables. Only one-half of the fruits offered may be 100% juice, because whole and cut-up fruits have more fiber.
>
> ▸ **Protein foods:** Meat, poultry, fish, dry beans, peas, eggs, nuts, and seeds provide many nutrients, including protein and iron. Portion sizes are based on the nutrition needs of children in various grade groups. School meals also allow cheese, tofu, and yogurt to count as the meat/meat alternate in the school lunch.
>
> Source: US Department of Agriculture. MyPlate guide to school lunch for families. https://www.fns.usda.gov/sites/default/files/tn/SL_Infographic_81216a.pdf. Published August 2016. Accessed October 31, 2017.

- Add a piece of fruit to your child's lunch sack and perhaps a bag of pretzels.
- Pack a small water bottle for him too.
- Work with your school wellness committee to improve school lunch selection.
- Find out what the policies are for food sold at school or at after-school events and advocate for healthy snacks and beverages.
- Work with your parent-teacher association to help get healthy food in schools.
- Advocate with your school board for healthier school meals and snacks.

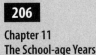

After-school Snacks

Once your child gets home from school, he might head straight for the cupboard or refrigerator and look for something to munch on. Have some healthy snacks for him to choose from—raw vegetables with nonfat dip, fresh fruit, whole-grain crackers, air-popped popcorn, unsalted pretzels, or baked tortillas with salsa. Keep the ice cream, cookies, and cakes out of reach—or better yet, out of the house altogether (reserve them for special occasions). By limiting access to snack foods like these, you're helping your child win the battle against weight gain.

Food Temptations

Meanwhile, stay alert for other potential stumbling blocks to healthy eating. For example, your school-aged child may sometimes exchange food with friends, giving up the sandwich and fruit that you've packed for him and trading them for a bag of potato chips. After school, if he's spending time at a playmate's home, he might be snacking there on candy rather than an apple. In short, even if you've done a good job of educating your child on making nutritious food choices, he'll face plenty of temptations, almost on a daily basis. (See the Eating Meals Away From Home section later in this chapter.)

Also, remember that you're a role model in this process, so make healthy food choices for yourself as well as the rest of the family. Even though school-aged children are busier than ever, make an effort to find time for family meals as often as possible. When all of you sit down at the dining room table together, it's a perfect opportunity for every family member to describe his or her day and for the family to grow closer.

YOUR CHILD AND BULLYING

Sadly, bullying is prevalent at all ages, and children are being teased for being a certain size, race, ethnicity, gender, or other aspects that may make them a target. Bullying is a serious issue and needs to be addressed as soon as possible. Your child may not tell you that he is being bullied, so you need to keep communication open and be on the alert. Here are some tips to help you identify if your child is experiencing bullying or if you already know he is being bullied:

▸ Keep the lines of communication open. Nonjudgmental listening and being available at times your child wants to talk are important for creating an environment in which he can tell you if he is encountering problems.

▸ Bullying can have physical signs as well as show up as altered behavior. Look for scrapes and bruises, change in behavior, anxiety about attending school, fear of riding the bus, anxiety of being with peers, sadness, depression, and other behavioral changes.

▸ Notify the school in writing of any bullying complaints immediately.

▸ Never ignore or downplay the importance of such complaints. Do not attempt to confront the bully or his or her family directly.

▸ Keep a record of incidents and always follow up with school administrators.

▸ Report to authorities and advocacy groups as needed to help navigate the situation.

▸ Explore other activities outside school to broaden peer groups, finding something your child can feel good about and excel in.

▸ Discuss safety plans for your child if he feels unsafe or harassed.

▸ Ensure that your child understands that it is not his fault and he has nothing to be ashamed of.

Consult StopBullying.gov (**https://www.stopbullying.gov**) for more information on bullying.

Source: StopBullying.gov

The Pediatrician's Role

During your child's school-age years, he may see your pediatrician for routine well-child examinations about every 1 to 2 years. If your child has obesity, you may need to schedule appointments more often. Your pediatrician can regularly calculate his BMI and help guide your family toward better nutrition and more physical activity as well as help you troubleshoot if your child is having difficulties in one health-related area or another.

If your child has a BMI greater than the 95th percentile, your pediatrician may do 3 things.

1 **Your pediatrician will ask a series of questions to find out if your child has been affected by any obesity-related health conditions.** These are medical problems that result from the effect of obesity on other body systems, such as the lungs, heart, liver, and bones. Your pediatrician may ask about headaches, vision problems, difficulty breathing normally or with exercise, stomach problems, constipation, urination, and pain or discomfort with your child's joints, especially his hips and knees. Your pediatrician will also ask about your child's mood, feelings, and depression and if he has been bullied or teased. Your pediatrician will perform a physical examination. It is important for your child's well-being that your pediatrician understands your child's health status as completely as possible. If necessary, your pediatrician will order laboratory studies based on your child's history and the physical examination.

② **Your pediatrician will want to know as much detail as possible about your child's lifestyle, family eating and activity patterns, and family and cultural traditions that affect nutrition and activity.** (See the diet and activity record in Table 9-1.) Treatment of obesity in children starts with taking a close look at what they are eating and what kind of activity and inactivity they engage in every day, as well as understanding their sleep patterns.

③ **Instilling change is challenging, and your pediatrician may use something called motivational interviewing to help you identify the goals you have for your child.** Motivational interviewing is a way of having a conversation that allows you to focus on what is most important to you and your child and helps you and your child pick which changes you feel most motivated to tackle.

The next sections will give you some ideas of an approach to healthy eating and activity to help you pick a starting place for your child for a healthy lifestyle change.

It Takes a Family: Nutrition + Fitness

What was your initial reaction when you realized that your child needed to control his weight? In that situation, many parents find themselves thinking, "I've got to put him on a diet." After all, in a culture in which thinness seems to be the name of the game and Americans just can't get their fill of diet books, you might instinctively think that the solution rests with the latest weight-loss fad, even though these diets are rarely designed with growing children or good nutrition in mind.

No matter what some diet gurus proclaim, calorie counting and exercising to the point of fatigue are *not* the answer, particularly for children. In fact, restricting calories in a growing child could pose risks to his health. You shouldn't do so unless your child's pediatrician recommends and supervises those efforts.

So what's the answer? As we've emphasized throughout this book, consistently good nutrition, meal after meal, is a foundation for a healthy childhood. Rather than becoming preoccupied with weight-loss goals, you should focus instead on a wholesome lifestyle for everyone in your family, no matter what each member weighs.

Establish some routines to your family's eating—3 well-thought-out meals and 1 snack a day. If you take steps to minimize the junk food in your family's diet, eliminate sugared beverages like soft drinks, pay attention to portion sizes, and add some physical activity to the mix, your heavy child *will* grow up to have a healthy lifestyle and increase their chances of achieving a healthy weight.

In preparing foods high in nutritional value, build the family meals around selections like

- Fresh fruits and vegetables
- Whole-grain cereals and bread
- Low-fat or nonfat dairy products, like milk, yogurt, and cheeses
- Lean and skinless meats, including chicken, turkey, fish, and lean hamburger

The basics of good nutrition really aren't that complicated. It means choosing or preparing a grilled chicken sandwich instead of a high-fat cheeseburger. Refer to Chapter 2, as well as the government's online ChooseMyPlate.gov (**https://www.choosemyplate.gov**), if you need a refresher course on the types of foods that should be part of your child's diet each day. Portion sizes at this age should be less than that of an adult-sized serving. Remember that when you're in the kitchen, choose cooking methods that involve a minimal amount of fat, relying primarily on broiling, roasting, and steaming.

Eating Meals Away From Home

On average, school-aged children eat at least one meal a day away from home. Often, that meal is at school or friends' homes, and you don't always know what and how much your child is eating. No wonder most parents have heard their children griping that friends or classmates have some privilege, experience, or food that they don't.

It can be frustrating, but never lose sight of the fact that you're in charge of your home environment. As the person in charge, you are making the food menu, shopping, and meal preparation decisions. At the same time, you are also engaging your child in a dialogue about healthy food choices, introducing new foods, and providing him with age-appropriate explanations of why your family is making nutritional changes. Keep in mind that while an 11-year-old can comprehend much more about the need to improve the food choices on your dinner table than a 6-year-old, most children understand when you tell them that "our entire family is making changes so we can be as healthy as possible."

Now, what can you do when your school-aged child is away from home? As you know, you'll lose some control over what he eats when he spends time at friends' houses. He might be able to choose soft drinks instead of milk there, or cookies rather than an apple or orange. At a fast-food restaurant with friends, he might feel peer pressure or be tempted to choose a supersized burger and fries rather than a smaller hamburger and salad. But you can enlist the help of the parents of your child's friends—ask for their support in keeping unhealthy snacks away from your child, making it easier for your child to make better choices. The same goes for other adults with whom your child spends time, including child care providers and grandparents.

Sure, your child might complain, "Everyone else has cookies in their lunch bags. Why do you give me an orange instead?" Or you may hear the common refrain, "It's not fair!"

Well, he's right—it may not seem fair. Remind him, "We're trying to eat better in our family because we want to be healthier as a family." If your child is old enough to understand, try accentuating the positive. For example, "You're a good student—you inherited that from our family. You also know that our family has trouble with weight, and we have to take care of that so we can stay as healthy as possible."

As these changes are made, let your child feel some sense of control over the situation. Let him make choices among many healthy alternatives.

Encourage him to lend a hand in the kitchen, helping you prepare a meal now and then. Explain why milk is a better selection than soda and why a pear is healthier than a candy bar. Remind your child that he can have the cookies or chips that he craves on occasion, although not as an everyday event. At the same time, introduce him to healthier alternatives that he may develop a taste for, such as low-fat baked tortilla chips rather than higher fat potato chips.

Involve Your Child in Planning and Preparing

One way of helping your child develop lifelong healthy habits and skills is to involve him in meal planning and preparation. You may want to have him help plan a meal he thinks the family will like. Helping to make a shopping list, picking out the ingredients at the grocery store, helping to chop and bake, and setting the table are all ways he can make a nutritious meal for everyone!

Making Fitness a Way of Life

Some school-aged children can't wait to get home from school, stake out a place on the couch, and spend the rest of the afternoon and evening watching TV. Physical activity is just not on their radar screens, at least not by choice.

Not surprisingly, children who fit this profile may be on a slippery slope to a life of struggling with their weight. There are a lot of them. Studies have shown that only one-quarter of school-aged children get the recommended 60 minutes of activity every day.

During your child's school-age years, your goal should be not only to get your child moving but to turn exercise into a lifelong habit. Just as in younger age groups, free play and recreational activities should make up most of the physical activity for the school-aged child. Children 6 to 10 years of age who want to play organized sports should be in ones that are of short duration, have limited rules, and allow some free play. Older school-aged

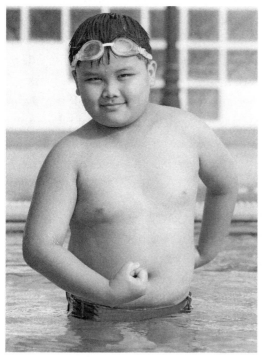

children can choose to get involved in organized sports, including Little League, youth soccer, a martial arts class, or community basketball, hockey, or football leagues. At this age team sports should be fun and geared toward participation and building team skills. However, group activities like these aren't for everyone. Some children feel self-conscious about participating in team sports and are much more comfortable getting their exercise in unstructured settings. For them, free play on the playground, ice-skating, in-line skating, bowling, or even running through sprinklers is more comfortable. Let your child choose something that he finds enjoyable, and once he discovers it, encourage him to make it a regular part of life. At the same time, limit TV watching or time spent on the computer or playing video games to no more than 1 hour a day. Studies have shown that the more time children devote to watching TV, the more likely they are to consume unhealthy foods that contribute to weight gain.

What if your child insists that he doesn't want to do any physical activity? Explain that it's important and might even be fun to find a new activity. Try to find activities that fit the family's budget and time commitments and have him choose among several options. Some children might prefer to go with a friend or parent. Be creative and emphasize participation, not competition. To help your school-aged youngster become physically active, recruit the entire family to participate. Let your child know that all of you, parents and siblings alike, are in his corner, and even if he has rarely exercised before, he can start now with the entire family's support. Go for family bike rides (with everyone wearing a helmet). Swim together at the Y. Take brisk walks. Learn to cross-country ski. Sign up for golf lessons. It is also important to think of different types of physical activity that take into account the different times of the day that he will be physically active, as well as different activities for various weather and times of the year that he can remain active throughout.

You can even do activities of daily living together, such as household chores. Spend a Saturday afternoon cleaning the house or raking leaves. No matter what you choose, regular activity not only burns calories but also strengthens your child's cardiovascular system, builds strong bones and muscles, and increases flexibility. It can also diffuse stress, help him learn teamwork and sportsmanship, boost his self-esteem, and improve his overall sense of well-being.

Throughout this book, we've emphasized the concerns that the American Academy of Pediatrics (AAP) has with children watching TV, particularly in excessive amounts. When it comes to children's programming, the primary goal of the networks is to market the products of advertisers—from toys to junk food—to children. Younger children, in particular, including those in the early elementary school years, cannot distinguish between programs and the commercials that surround them; nor do they fully understand that the intent of advertising is to get them (and their parents) to buy products in supermarkets and toy stores.

The AAP strongly supports improvements in the overall quality of children's programming and encourages parents to limit the amount of time that their kids spend in front of the TV.

Challenges in Maintaining Healthy Lifestyle Changes

Sneaking Food

Imagine thinking that your child is making all the right nutritional choices, and then discovering a bag of potato chips or cookies in his dresser drawer. Or just when you think that he's sticking to a healthy eating routine, you discover that the snack foods that were on a high shelf in the kitchen cupboard have "mysteriously" vanished. In fact, plenty of school-aged children sneak food, often believing (or at least hoping) that they'll never get caught. Quite often, they seem surprised when they're confronted about their behavior. In fact, they may deny it at first before finally admitting that they've been doing it. Children may sneak food for a variety of reasons. Perhaps eating can ease the stress they're experiencing over upcoming examinations or because they're being teased or bullied at school. Maybe they just want to feel a greater sense of control over their environment. When you become aware of sneaking behaviors, it is important to keep your own disappointment or anger in check.

Here are some tips to help get your child back on track.

- Let your child know that you've discovered that he's been sneaking food, and calmly talk with him about why he's doing it. Remember to ask and then listen. You can then remind him about the family goal of healthier eating.
- Offer to help your child find other strategies to address his hunger aside from food. Suggest positive ways for him to respond when he feels that he absolutely has to eat something, even when it's not time for a regular meal or snack. For example, he can
  - Ride his bicycle.
  - Go for a walk with you.
  - Kick a soccer ball with a friend.
  - Read a book.
  - Go for a run.
  - Finish a puzzle.
  - Help out with household chores.
- You may want to set up a system that gives your child points or stars that can be redeemed for rewards when he asks for food rather than sneaking it. He might earn points that he can accumulate for rewards like a game or new piece of sports equipment, a special outing, or those special sneakers. Talk about these rewards in advance, and stick to them. For many children, this system can be very effective in minimizing sneaking.
- Never punish a child for eating the wrong foods, even if this occurs soon after you've explicitly instructed your child not to do so. Removing privileges may be hard to resist, but resist them. In a year or two your child may become more naturally interested in controlling his unhealthy eating impulses. Do not allow negative strategies this year to jeopardize future possibilities of success.
- Remember, the best way to eliminate sneaking food is to remove the most tempting snack foods from the household; this reduces temptation and benefits the whole family.
- Having regularly scheduled meals and snacks can also help reduce long stretches of hunger and the temptation to sneak.

Separate Households and Eating Routines

Children often find themselves splitting their time between households. They may be alternating weeks or days with parents who are divorced and living in different households. They may be spending every afternoon with grandparents or summers with other relatives. It is important for families to be on the same page as often as possible with regard to providing healthy eating and activity. Here are some tips that may help.

- If possible, family members may want to visit your child's pediatrician together to talk about eating, activity, and screen time goals. Even though families are separated, the same principles of family-based healthy lifestyle change apply.
- If you are the one who is initiating a healthy lifestyle plan for your child, it is important to discuss your child's health and need to improve his nutrition and physical activity with everyone taking care of him. Sharing information from your pediatrician, goals and strategies for change, and the hope that everyone can be consistent is critical.
- One technique to help keep track of healthy eating and activity is to use a small notebook or tablet that everyone can use to record meals, snacks, beverages, activity, and screen time so you can understand what is happening when your child is away. Clearly, this works best if approached in a nonjudgmental way and records are used to discuss goals and strategies with your pediatrician.
- If other family members are reluctant to participate, concentrate on your own home environment and family routines. It can be difficult to know that others are offering your child foods and activities that you are working hard to change, but keep calm and remember that if you are providing a role model of a healthy lifestyle, your child will benefit in the long run.

Your child may want to have a discussion with family members themselves and ask for healthy snacks and opportunities to be active. If so, be supportive of your child taking the initiative whichever way the discussion turns out.

What Would You Do?

You have just picked your daughter up from after-school care. It's 5:00 pm and you want to get home and start cooking dinner. You get stuck in traffic, and after she has told you all about school, she starts to complain of being hungry. You had planned to cook a meal—you bought the ingredients and planned a healthy menu that morning—but now you are feeling stressed. You start to think of all the things you and your daughter have to do before bedtime and the short amount of time you have to do them.

- Cook dinner.
- Clean up.
- Get homework done.
- Help her with the science project she is working on for later that week.
- Try to fit in that workout you promised to do with her.
- Get clothes ready for school tomorrow.
- Pack her lunch.

You know you are running out of time and may feel that your only choices are

- Skip the workout.
- Order out for dinner.
- Give her lunch money for tomorrow.
- Put off the science project to another night.
- Let her stay up a little longer to get her homework done.

Handling Inevitable Stress

After-school time can feel like you are running a marathon. Here are some tips to lessen the stress and still keep your healthy lifestyle goals.

- Stress is a part of life; keep 6 or 7 frozen meals that you have prepared in advance in the freezer. Pull these out on your most stressful days.

- A sandwich, soup or salad, piece of fruit, and a glass of milk is a meal. On days when you know you are running out of time, give yourself a break and make this as a quick way to prepare dinner. There's also more time to talk to each other and less cleanup!
- Have your child pack his own lunch while you are getting dinner ready. Store the ingredients in an easily accessible place and work together. Two meals are prepared at the same time!
- Kids often need a physical break between school and homework. If there is a way to get outside and play, they can burn off some steam while you are getting dinner on the table.
- This is where having a screen time schedule can really help. Decide on what and at what time your child can watch his show or play his game. It's often hard to pull a child away from a screen, so it is easier if homework and chores come first.

Goal Setting: Improve Your Child's and Family's Nutrition

After reading this chapter, you may have a goal in mind, such as reducing portion sizes, healthier snacking, or limiting or eliminating sugared beverages. Keep in mind that your goal should be aimed at helping your child but will often include the whole family in the change process. A few points about what makes a good goal include

- **The goal should be specific.** For example, instead of saying your child will cut down on sugary drinks, a more specific goal would be, "Instead of 3 sugary drinks per day, cut down to 1 sugary drink per day."
- **The goal should be important to you and your child.** It takes energy to work on a goal, and your chances of success are better if your goal is meaningful to you. For example, if your child's aunt just developed diabetes, cutting down on sugary treats may be on everyone's to-do list and be a goal the whole family can get behind.

■ **The goal should be something you think you can really do.** Taking small steps is important here. Instead of saying, "We will walk 2 miles per day," you can start with, "We will walk around the block as a family after dinner each day." Achieving a goal is satisfying and you can always increase the difficulty level of the next goal you set.

Here are 10 steps for setting, keeping track of, and troubleshooting a goal.

1 **Identify your child's dilemma or issue that needs change.** For example, say the issue is, "My child eats too much fast food." Ask, "How can my child and family address this?" There may be more than one answer. In our example, you could

- Limit fast food meals from 3 to 1 per week.
- Choose water or milk, salad instead of fries, and a regular burger instead of an extra-large one when you do eat out.
- Split a meal with another sibling or parent when eating fast food.
- Eliminate fast food and spend the money on a family activity.

2 **Pick a goal that is meaningful for you and your family,** such as limiting fast food if you know your family has a history of heart disease.

3 **Make sure the goal is doable for you and your family.** For example, limiting fast-food meals to 1 per week from 3 may be an easier way to start that completely eliminating fast food.

4 **Decide how you will accomplish your goal,** such as

- Plan ahead and choose the day of the week you will eat out.
- Plan simple family meals for the days you decided to eat at home.
- Keep track of when you eat out on the calendar.

5 **Check in with yourself.** In a week or two see if you were able to accomplish the goal.

 Troubleshoot the goal. If you are having trouble, see if you can figure out why. For example

- Your family ate out an extra time because you had a very busy day.

- Your child insisted you have fast food for dinner twice in one week.
- You had an activity to go to and it was easier to pick up a fast-food meal on the way.

7 **See if you can troubleshoot a solution.** For example, if the problem was that your child had an activity to go to and you drove through and got fast food, you could instead

- Eat an earlier meal before the activity.
- Pack a meal to eat in the car.
- Pack a snack to tide everyone over and cook a meal when you get home.

8 **Check back with yourself in a week or two and see if you were able to accomplish the goal** of having only 1 fast-food meal per week.

9 **Keep going until you have made this a routine.**

10 **Then pick another goal,** maybe one about exercising or reducing screen time, and start again.

Key Points to Remember

1 Your child needs your support more than ever as he encounters various environments and temptations at school, activities with friends, and the community.

2 Time becomes even more scarce, and after-school time is at a premium. Meal planning, routines, and schedules for play can help make the most of this limited resource.

3 Family activities are important, and weekends can be a great time to try a new sport, physical activity, or hobby together.

4 Setting specific goals that are meaningful and doable for you and your family is the way to make progress on achieving a healthy lifestyle.

5 Stressful times happen for everyone. Planning for these times by having extra meals in the freezer, simplifying meals, and working in physical activity can get you through tough times until you can get back to your routines.

Resources

Active healthy living: prevention of childhood obesity through increased physical activity. *Pediatrics.* 2006;117(5):1834–1842

National Physical Activity Plan Alliance Report Card Research Advisory Committee. *The 2014 United States Report Card on Physical Activity for Children & Youth.* American College of Sports Medicine Web site. https://www.acsm.org/docs/default-source/other-documents/nationalreportcard_longform_final-for-web(2).pdf?sfvrsn=0). Accessed October 31, 2017

Resnicow K, Harris D, Wasserman R, et al. Advances in motivational interviewing for pediatric obesity: results of the Brief Motivational Interviewing to Reduce Body Mass Index Trial and future directions. *Pediatr Clin North Am.* 2016;63(3):539–562

Chapter 12

The Adolescent Years

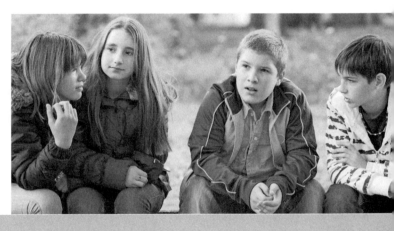

If there's a teenager in your family, you don't need to be reminded about the many challenges of parenting an adolescent, guiding her from childhood into adulthood. If your teenager has obesity added to the mix of challenges, it might seem as though your parenting skills are constantly being put to the test.

Perhaps you've already spoken to your teenager's pediatrician about just how high the stakes are for your adolescent and her present and future health. A teenager with obesity not only faces health risks today, such as diabetes, liver disease, lipid problems, hypertension, and sleep apnea, but she also has about an 80% chance of becoming an adult with obesity. To complicate matters, you probably feel that you have less control than ever over the factors that are contributing to your teenager's excess weight. This is a good time to help her develop the knowledge and skills to make the transition to her own healthy decision-making as a young adult. After all, she's probably spending less time at home than she used to, limiting your opportunities to prepare meals and encourage her to exercise. No wonder so many parents in your situation worry that the weight issue is largely beyond their influence. At times, you might find yourself thinking, "She eats so many meals away from home; how can I possibly have an effect anymore?"

That's certainly not the case.

Yes, your teenager is much more independent than she was 5 or 10 years ago, but you're still a very important person in her life, and it's essential that you stay connected. It's true that your involvement may no longer be the 24/7 hands-on role that you played in the past, but you can help guide her toward the independent decision-making she will need as an adult. You need to stay an active participant in her life and be there to help her build the skills and nurture her decision-making and behaviors that will transition her into a lifetime of healthy eating and regular physical activity.

The Parent's Role

Your Changing Role as a Parent

Your teenager is a different person than she once was. As an adolescent, she may not be capable of assuming adult responsibilities quite yet, but as she has grown and matured, she's now much more able to understand the implications and consequences of having obesity. As a result, you should address the issue of weight management differently than you once did.

When her weight is concerned, you will need to engage her in conversation about her health, her feelings, and thoughts about struggling with her weight in a world that's often unfriendly to heavy people.

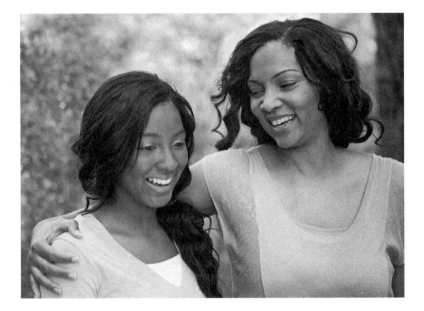

Beginning the Conversation: An Action Plan

- **Initiate the dialogue.** Asking your teen if she is worried about her health or weight is a good way to start. You can talk about health problems in the family, especially if others have struggled with weight issues or obesity-related diseases, like type 2 diabetes, and let your teen that know you are worried about her health too. Although this may motivate you, your teen may be much more concerned about immediate effects of her weight. Asking your teen if her weight is affecting her in any way may bring up issues, like fitting into clothes, wanting to look like the other girls, or having trouble keeping up in physical education. The important thing here is to *listen*.

- **Ask about the future.** If your teen is already concerned about her weight, you may ask, "What do you think will happen if your weight keeps going up?" Don't expect her to respond by saying, "Well, I might get diabetes or high blood pressure, and I don't want that to happen." But she may open up and begin talking about her frustration about being able to lose weight, her concerns about her body image, and what her classmates might be saying about the way she looks. This is an opening to offer your support.

- **Ask how you can help.** In the process, let your adolescent know that despite her growing independence, you're still her parent and you'll still be there when she needs you. A question that often opens up dialogue is asking your teen how you can best help her. She may surprise you by saying to get rid of the sugary drinks, go to healthier restaurants when the family eats out, or even ask her brother not to bring home junk food.

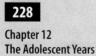
- If she isn't sure, you can say, "Let's continue to work on your weight together," and then offer some suggestions, such as
  - "We can go on family hikes on the weekends."
  - "Let's go grocery shopping together and help make healthy lunches for school ahead of time."
  - "We can go on bike rides."
  - "I'll continue to prepare nutritious meals when you're home, and there'll be plenty of healthy choices in the refrigerator for snacking."

  And then listen to her response.
- **Keep listening.** Let her know that you know how hard it can be to manage healthy eating and activity when she is away from home. You can say, "I'm always available to talk with you about any problems you may have keeping to a healthy eating and activity plan."
- **Support your adolescent's healthy choices.** At times, you will want to give your adolescent some space. Make suggestions, gently offer advice, but also give your teenager some space to make choices on her own, and let her know that you trust her to make good ones. Sure, there will be times when she doesn't make the best decisions, but at her age, putting more control in her hands works better than saying, "Here's what you need to do—turn off the TV and go outside right now!" or "I don't care where your friends like to go—you've got to stop eating at fast-food restaurants!"
- **Keep the dialogue open.** Ask questions like
  - "What's been the hardest part about managing your weight this week?"
  - "What can I do to help?"
  - "What can we think of together that will keep you moving in the right direction?"

- **Discuss your role.** Explain to your teenager that, in a sense, you've become something akin to her coach. Remind her that even the most elite athletes need coaches, and it isn't a sign of weakness or failure. Don't offer advice at every turn, or she's liable to shut the door without even listening. Just let her know that you're available to talk and give guidance when she wants it. By all means, create a home environment that's conducive to success.

- **Look at your own behavior.** The bottom line is that your role is changing, and that means posing some questions to yourself too. For example, are you asking your teenager to make changes in her eating or activity level that you're not doing yourself? Are you sabotaging her efforts to eat healthy by keeping junk food in the pantry or baking holiday cookies and leaving them out where she can't help but be tempted? Are you framing your comments to your child in a supportive manner? For instance, rather than asking, "Why are you so lazy when it comes to exercising?" you could say, "Why don't we get the entire family to go play tennis this afternoon?"

- **Don't let up on family support.** Even though your teenager is much more capable of taking the weight issue into her own hands, she can still use all the support that's offered. You and your other family members should join forces to become your teenager's most loyal support team. Let your adolescent know that the entire family will provide what she needs to help her make wise decisions about her weight. Sometimes, teenagers may act as though their friends are much more important to them than family. You and the rest of your family will continue to be much more indispensable to her than she's sometimes willing to admit.

The Pediatrician's Role

How Your Teen's Pediatrician Can Help

- **Encourage the conversation.** Sometimes teens do not want to talk about their weight. It can be an uncomfortable topic for them, and they may not open up quickly—or at all. If you are having trouble talking with your teen about her weight, your teen's pediatrician can help get the ball rolling. If it is time for a checkup, your pediatrician will be discussing height, weight, and body mass index (BMI) just like your pediatrician has been doing all along, opening the door to talk with your teen about her health choices.

- Don't be surprised if the conversation starts to be aimed at your teen. Watch and see how this goes. Many times you can use this as a jumping-off point for continuing the discussion at home.

- If you become concerned and want to talk about your teen's weight between well checkups, you can always schedule a visit with your teen's pediatrician to do just that. Just be sure you and your teen have discussed the reason for the visit before you both get to the appointment. If you want to talk by phone with your pediatrician beyond scheduling a visit, it is preferable to include your teen on the call. The message here is that you are in this together.

- **Evaluate her health and behaviors.** Adolescence is a crucial time to set the stage for the independence of young adulthood. Your pediatrician will evaluate your teen for obesity-related conditions and risky health behaviors. They may want to do this in private, and that can be an important step in the transition to your adolescent's self-care. However, also having a family-based discussion is critical to setting attainable nutrition and activity goals and making sure the family can provide needed support and all be on the same page.

- **Assess the environment.** Peers, school, and the neighborhood can all be powerful influences over your adolescent's health behaviors. Your pediatrician will want to understand what is happening in the environment that surrounds your adolescent. The pediatrician may want to discuss these external factors in private, as well.
- **Assess and understand your adolescent's mood and mental health.** Adolescence can be a time of increased stress, escalated expectations, and increased body consciousness. Adding obesity to the mix can often result in difficulties with anxiety, self-esteem, or depression. It is important for your teen's pediatrician to understand just how your adolescent is thinking and feeling and be able to offer support and treatment if needed.

A Proper Diet for Your Growing Teenager

Ask the average adolescent to describe her perfect meal, and she's liable to say, "A double cheeseburger with large fries," or maybe, "Pepperoni pizza—as many slices as I can fit on my plate."

For a teenager with a weight problem, however, those may not be the optimal choices, as popular as they may be. No matter how your own teenager would describe her ideal meal, there's no doubt that nutrition is crucial at this time of life. She's going through puberty and growing rapidly, and, particularly if she's heavy, she needs to become conscientious about eating a healthy diet.

- Teenagers need to eat a variety of nutritional foods and rely more often on fruits and vegetables, whole grains, low-fat dairy, and lean meat. That means ordering or selecting grilled chicken sandwiches more often than a cheeseburger and consuming meals with vegetables and fruits as well as pasta, rice, and a variety of other foods.
- Serving sizes for teenagers should be about the same as they are for adults. Rather than putting serving dishes on the dining room table and letting family members help themselves, prepare everyone's plate away from the table to keep from tempting your adolescent to help herself to seconds—and thirds.

For more information on meal planning, see Chapter 2. As you use the information in Chapter 2 as a guide, there are some obstacles that your teenager may face when trying to eat in ways that support effective weight management.

Skipping Meals

Adolescents are renowned for skipping meals—most often, breakfast and/or lunch—and this can throw their entire nutritional programs off-kilter. According to a recent study, about 43% of boys and girls aged 12 to 19 years said that they didn't eat breakfast on school mornings.

Your teenager may tell you that she prefers to sleep a little later, even if it means leaving for school on an empty stomach.

Even if your adolescent believes that those extra minutes of sleep are just too precious to sacrifice, there are still ways to keep her well-nourished. Why not spend a few minutes in the evening preparing a breakfast-to-go for the following day? Perhaps you can slice a bagel that can be quickly toasted in the morning (use peanut butter rather than cream cheese as a spread). Hard-boil an egg that can be eaten in the car. Put some nuts and raisins in a plastic bag for her to nibble on. Let her eat a container of yogurt or an apple. All these choices may be enough to tide her over until she's able to sit down for a well-balanced meal later in the day. Encourage her to take over as she gets into a routine and to ask if she needs help.

Snacking

For the average teenager, snacking seems to be a way of life. In fact, one-quarter of the caloric intake of adolescents comes from snacks. Yet too often, their preference of snack foods is a little suspect. Given the choice, many teenagers would rather grab a handful of potato chips than grapes.

However, when it's time for a snack (which, for many adolescents, is most of the time), they'll reach for what's available. For that reason, make an effort to keep your refrigerator and pantry stocked with healthy snacks. That means choosing foods like low-fat cheeses, nonfat frozen yogurt, applesauce, or air-popped popcorn.

Eating Away From Home

Because teenagers eat many of their meals outside the home, adult caregivers aren't there to keep an eye on what they're putting on their plates. Not surprisingly, some of their choices fall short of what they should be.

At school, some adolescents will settle for a stop at the vending machine at lunch and consume a bag of cookies and a soft drink before their next classes. If they're eating at a fast-food restaurant or a pizza shop with friends, they may decide that fitting in with their peers is more important than making healthy food selections.

When your teenager is away from home, you can't reasonably ask her to always avoid fast-food restaurants, particularly when that's where her friends go on Saturday night. But you can ask her something like, "Can you think of anything you could order besides a large hamburger, large fries, and a shake?" Remind her that it doesn't have to be an all-or-nothing proposition, and if she's open to suggestions, perhaps you can guide her toward making healthier decisions ("How about choosing a chicken sandwich, plus a salad with low-fat dressing?"). If she's going out for pizza with friends, remind her that while she can certainly have a slice of pizza, why not balance it with a salad? She might also develop a taste for thin-crust vegetarian pizza instead of thick-crust pepperoni pizza with double cheese.

Remember, this is a learning process, and you can't expect your teenager to always make healthy choices. Over time, she'll get better at it. Also, remind her that when she's out with friends, she doesn't have to eat the entire time. Often, just hanging out with her buddies is enough. For example, ask your adolescent, "Can you suggest something else to do with your friends besides going to a restaurant? Maybe you could go bowling or to the batting cages?"

On the other hand, she might tell you, "I'm going to feel funny if I don't eat something when all my friends are ordering food." She may be right, but she can still be more selective in the food she buys and puts on her plate.

The Lure of Fad Diets

Sometimes, it seems as though teenaged girls and boys talk as much about diets as any other topic of conversation. Particularly if they're preoccupied with their weight, they can hardly wait to share the newest quick-fix eating plan they've found, latching onto one crazy diet or another with little attention paid to how poor its nutritional value might be. One month, they might be trying a low-carbohydrate diet; the next, a high-carbohydrate diet. Or they'll become hooked on a grapefruit diet one week and a fruit-free diet the following week. They probably won't stay on any of them for very long, but as they hopscotch from one to another, good nutrition may fall by the wayside. These diets are usually too restrictive and too unhealthy. With weight loss in mind, they won't work over the long run either. Any change in diet should be discussed with and approved by your teen's pediatrician, so everyone is on the same page and can report on progress and/or signs of concern.

Endless Hunger Pangs

Does it seem like your teenager is always hungry? Since she entered and began moving through puberty, have you noticed that the refrigerator and kitchen cupboard doors are getting a real workout, hour after hour, day after day? Does it seem like shortly after a trip to the supermarket, it's time to go back because the cupboards are becoming bare again?

As part of adolescence, your child's appetite may be soaring off the charts as her need for calories escalates to support normal growth spurts. Nevertheless, despite her constant craving for food, you and your teen don't have to give up the battle against her weight problem.

Here's a basic principle to keep in mind: As long as you're providing your adolescent with well-balanced nutrition and high-quality foods, and she's eating 3 reasonably sized meals per day plus 1 to 2 snacks, her weight should be just fine. If she's still telling you with regularity that she's absolutely famished, and if it's also a time when she's growing, check with your pediatrician to monitor her BMI and make sure she is eating nutritious food, not a couple of candy bars, at meals and snacks.

Breaking a Sweat for Weight Loss

Many children seem to be in constant motion in their early years. All that activity often comes to an end in adolescence, as the time and opportunities for physical activity begin to wane. At many middle and high schools, physical education programs have been curtailed or completely eliminated. Add to that the demands of after-school activities such as music lessons and school plays, part-time jobs, homework, and the availability of television (TV), video games, and computers, and many adolescents complain that there simply isn't time to be active.

Nearly every teenager can find some form of activity that she enjoys and is willing to do regularly, whether it's throwing a ball with a neighborhood friend or joining an evening basketball league at the YMCA. Don't forget sports that your teenager can develop a love for that can last for decades, including golf, tennis, skating, and skiing.

What if your adolescent resists doing any kind of activity? Don't give up hope. If she seems glued to the TV or computer, ask her, "What else can you do besides watch TV?" If she says, "I don't know," you might say, "Let's figure it out together." Sometimes, you can get her interested by saying, "Let's both sign up for an exercise class at the gym, like Zumba!"

Any form of movement is better than letting your child sit in front of a screen all afternoon. Start with little steps on getting her interested in an activity, even if doing so doesn't involve an overtly physical activity. Encourage her to volunteer at the senior center, or maybe she can join the choir at church. She can get a part-time job at the community recreation center, helping organize games for younger kids. Then slowly work toward seeing if there's a way to build some exercise into those seemingly sedentary activities. When given the choice to take the elevator or stairs, encourage her to take the stairs. If she's working at the recreation center, can she fit some walking into her required tasks?

Even if you often hear the complaint, "I don't have time to exercise," your teenager may actually have more time than she thinks. There are probably 15 or 20 minutes during her afternoon or evening when she's sitting in front of the computer and could shift gears and use some of that sedentary time for physical activity.

WHEN EATING GETS OUT OF CONTROL

If your teenager's attempts at sensible weight loss don't seem to be working, and she moves from one fad diet to another with nothing to show for it but a lot of anguish and frustration, she might ultimately join the ranks of many other adolescents by resorting to a dangerous lifestyle of an eating disorder, like bulimia nervosa. As their preoccupation with weight and body image intensifies, teenagers may start bingeing on food (often high-calorie junk food), consuming thousands of calories at a sitting, with seemingly no control over what they're doing. Once a bingeing episode has run its course, which could take an hour or two (or sometimes more), they purge themselves by self-induced vomiting or abusing laxatives or diuretics.

For most adolescents who have bulimia, these bingeing-and-purging cycles repeat themselves day after day. These teenagers eat emotionally, even when they're not hungry, typically trying to compensate for or cope with low self-esteem and feelings of inadequacy. They usually feel guilty and disgusted by what they're doing and often hide food in their dresser drawers or closets. They may become depressed or experience mood swings, and despite symptoms like swollen glands in their necks and erosion of their tooth enamel (which is associated with vomiting), they can't stop this cycle of emotional eating.

Millions of Americans have one type of eating disorder or another—not only bingeing and purging to avoid gaining weight but also under-eating or self-starvation (anorexia nervosa), as well as gorging on food without any purging involved in it. Although these eating problems affect primarily girls and women in their teens and twenties, some boys have these disorders as well. They can go undetected for years, with teenagers often planning their bingeing-and-purging episodes when no one else is home.

As a parent, be on the lookout for behaviors that lead you to suspect bulimia in your adolescent. Bulimia is a complex disorder; you can't assume that your teenager is going to outgrow it or that you can put a stop to the problem simply by telling her to quit. To support her recovery, you also need to seek professional help for her, and the earlier this intervention takes place, the better. Contact your teen's pediatrician, who will probably refer you to a specialist or treatment facility in this field. Your teenager may receive behavioral therapy (psychotherapy), nutritional counseling, and medications such as antidepressants to help her in the recovery process.

TEENS, DIET PILLS, AND SURGERY

Anyone who has tried to lose weight and keep it off, whether adolescents or adults, knows that it isn't easy. It takes commitment, perseverance, and plenty of patience.

In a society that values the quick fix, it's not surprising that some teenagers with obesity are turning to diet pills as the magic bullet to deliver them from the hard work of eating right and exercising regularly. Adolescents are asking their parents (and pediatricians) for weight-loss prescription drugs with increasing frequency. Or they're going to pharmacies on their own and buying over-the-counter diet pills that promise to melt away the pounds with no effort at all.

Your own teenager might be tempted to turn to these drugs, but it's unwise for her to do so. Let your adolescent know that there's no over-the-counter weight-loss drug that's been proven safe and effective for teenagers. Orlistat, a prescription weight-loss drug that blocks fat absorption in the intestine and has been approved by the US Food and Drug Administration for adolescents older than 12 years, is only useful in a few teens who meet strict criteria. This drug needs to be used under physician supervision to monitor the teen's nutrition and side effects of the drug. Weight control requires an effort over many months and even years, and none of the over-the-counter drugs were developed for long-term use.

Here's where you need to assert your parental authority. *Your teenager should not take diet pills.* There are safer ways to lose weight, and they're described throughout this book.

Now, what about weight-loss surgery? A small number of centers in the United States are performing surgery in adolescents with extreme obesity. Any surgical procedure carries risks, so these procedures should only be done in centers with adolescent weight management programs and an experienced team doing ongoing research into the long-term risks and benefits. Even though these operations can have dramatic weight-loss benefits, your teenager will still have to improve the way she eats and exercises in the aftermath of the surgery.

But for adolescents with severe obesity, weight-loss surgery may be the only option with a chance for success. Talk with your teen's pediatrician about the pros and cons of these operations, and if the doctor feels your adolescent is a candidate for the procedure, your pediatrician may refer you to an adolescent surgery program for an evaluation.

Wielding Your Influence: Coming Full Circle

If your teenager is like most others, she probably doesn't shop much in grocery stores. She leaves that to you, which allows you to remain the major influence on the foods she consumes in your home.

Whenever possible, encourage the family to have meals together. The fact is that families who eat together tend to have healthier diets than those whose members prepare something only for themselves or eat away from home a lot. Numerous studies have shown that boys and girls who frequently ate with their parents were more likely to eat the recommended number of servings of fruits and vegetables each day. Not only will your adolescent probably get better nutrition during these family meals, but you can also serve as a role model for the way she should be eating, even when she's not at home.

Helping Your Adolescent to Set a Goal to Achieve a Healthier Lifestyle

You may have a clear goal in mind for your adolescent, such as reducing portion sizes, managing screen time, or participating in physical activity. As you have probably seen by now, goal setting needs to be a joint effort. Clearly setting goals and keeping to them has a lot to do with motivation. Picking a goal that matters to your teen is a critical first step toward success. No matter where you start with setting a goal, you and your teen will be taking a positive step toward a healthier lifestyle.

Setting goals is a skill that parents and teens can develop together. Often this begins with a conversation with your pediatrician, who can help you identify possible goals and help you think about which ones are meaningful to you and your teen, as well as being something that you can accomplish. Here are 10 steps for setting a goal that will help you take the next step toward a healthier lifestyle.

Identify your teen's dilemma or issue that needs change. For example, say the issue is, "My teen has trouble making healthy choices when out with friends." Ask, "How can I help my teen address this?" There may be more than one answer. In our example, you could

- Agree to have a conversation before she goes out to go over possible healthy options, maybe by looking in advance at the restaurant menu.
- Rehearse responses to her friends if they insist that she eat more than she wants to.
- Discuss ordering a salad before or with the meal to help limit portions of unhealthy foods.
- Work on eliminating sugary drinks.

 Pick a goal that is meaningful to your teen, such as eliminating sugary drinks when eating out (you have already done this at home) because of her concern about her father's newly diagnosed diabetes.

❸ **Make sure the goal is doable for your teen.** For example, begin by having her limit herself to 1 sugary drink when she is eating out and then drinking water (her routine was to order 1–2 refills).

❹ **Decide how your teen will accomplish her goal,** such as writing down when she has a sugary beverage. With her agreement, you can help her by reminding her of her goal before she goes out and discussing how she did with her goal after she comes back.

❺ **Have your teen check in with herself and you.** In a week or two see if she was able to accomplish the goal.

❻ **Troubleshoot the goal.** If your teen is having trouble, see if you can help her figure out why. For example

- She forgot to write down how many sugary drinks she had each week.
- Peer pressure took over and she ordered refills of soda just like everyone else.
- She got caught up in the discussion and forgot to order water after her first soda.

See if you can help your teen troubleshoot a solution. For example, if the problem was that your teen got caught up in the discussion and forgot to order water, you could

- Suggest that she order water at the beginning of the meal with the soda, so it's right there.
- See if she will agree to a reminder from you about her goal, right before she leaves.
- If she is ready, suggest that she try ordering only water to make things simpler and to see how it feels to not have a sugary drink.

8 **Check back with your teen and you in a week or two and see if you were able to accomplish the goal** of having only 1 sugary drink with eating out.

9 **Keep going until your teen has made this a routine.**

10 **Then pick another goal,** maybe one about exercising or reducing screen time, **and start again.**

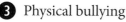
If Your Adolescent Is Being Bullied

Chapter 11 explained how bullying is becoming more prevalent among school-aged students, and this includes young adults. According to StopBullying.gov (**https://www.stopbullying.gov**), any unwanted or aggressive behavior toward another person can be considered a crime in some states. If your teen expresses any concerns about being bullied or knows someone being bullied or who is a bully, talk to her and consider talking to the school. You may need to report any incidents that require law enforcement or school officials.

According to StopBullying.gov, there are 3 types of bullying.

1 Verbal bullying

2 Social bullying

3 Physical bullying

- **Verbal bullying** is saying or writing mean things. Verbal bullying includes
  - Teasing
  - Name-calling
  - Inappropriate sexual comments
  - Taunting
  - Threatening to cause harm

- **Social bullying,** sometimes referred to as relational bullying, involves hurting someone's reputation or relationships. Social bullying includes
  - Leaving someone out on purpose
  - Telling other children not to be friends with someone
  - Spreading rumors about someone
  - Embarrassing someone in public

- **Physical bullying** involves hurting a person's body or possessions. Physical bullying includes
  - Hitting, kicking, or pinching
  - Spitting
  - Tripping or pushing
  - Taking or breaking someone's things
  - Making mean or rude hand gestures

Another form of bullying, cyberbullying, has become a very serious issue with the onset of new social media platforms. It includes harassment or any aggressive, unwanted behavior through the use of cell phone or online media. This includes, but is not limited to

- Text messages
- Voicemail
- E-mails
- Pictures or video
- Social media messages or posts

Parents can help prevent cyberbullying by having a conversation with their teen about safe online practices and responsible cell phone use. This may mean that you follow your teen online, have control settings on certain social networking platforms that limit your teen's capabilities, or opt in for notifications whenever your teen posts or leaves messages on the site. You may also consider whether specific phone apps or social networks are appropriate for your teen and determine when she can sign up.

Weight bias can be the cause of serious bullying of children and teens who have obesity. Resources addressing weight bias can be found at the UConn Rudd Center for Food Policy & Obesity Web site, **www.uconnruddcenter.org.**

Your Teen and Low Self-esteem

Struggling with weight is hard. Teens are exposed to external pressures to be thin and fit, media images that often portray people with obesity in a negative light, and criticism from family, friends, and peers. It is not hard to imagine how this would affect anyone's self-esteem. Here are some ideas that may help you understand your role in helping your teen achieve positive self-esteem.

- **Make sure your teen is not being teased or bullied** (see the If Your Adolescent Is Being Bullied section earlier in this chapter). This can occur not only with peers but family members and needs immediate intervention.
- **Stay positive.** When parents get anxious about their children, they often resort to nagging, pointing out the things they don't want them to do, and forgetting to recognize the positive things that are happening. Table 12-1 lists some personal strengths and includes space to list additional qualities. With your teen, discuss these strengths, add additional ones, and check the strengths you see in her. This can be an interesting discussion because you may see a strong point in your

teen that she does not recognize herself, which can provide a great opportunity to emphasize one of her positive qualities. Sometimes she will identify a strength you had overlooked, and this can be an opportunity for you to acknowledge this strong point. If there are strengths that you or she does not identify but she would like to develop, you can check these in the last column and work on finding ways to build on them.

Table 12-1. Strength Qualities		
Strengths	**Strengths I Currently Have**	**Strengths I Want to Develop**
Generosity		
Kindness		
Good at academics		
Creative		
A good friend to have		
Good at sports		

Combine this with goal setting and you may find that your teen feels more empowered to tackle moving to a healthier lifestyle.

■ Sometimes traditional sports or activities do not work for a teen struggling with weight and it helps to **try something different,** such as archery, scouting, chess, or art lessons. Any activity is better than no activity, and some of the more sedentary activities that get a teen away from screen time and involve peer interaction can be a first step to a more active lifestyle. This may provide a different peer group and a chance to develop a unique skill.

- **Be alert for signs of depression, anxiety, mood swings, and other behavior changes** that are worrisome, and talk with your teen's pediatrician right away to get a diagnosis and help.

What Would You Do?

Your whole family is invited to a family member's 16th birthday party. This is an evening event with a buffet dinner and cake and ice cream. Your teen is excited to go and spend time with her cousins. You arrive at the party and your adolescent heads straight for the buffet. The food does look delicious, and she helps herself to a heaping plateful of lasagna, chicken, and garlic bread and a cup of punch. As you circle back around the gathering you see she now has a large piece of cake and chocolate ice cream on her plate and is drinking a soda. Later in the evening you see her with her cousins snacking on chips and juice while playing a favorite video game. You feel a little desperate because you have been working diligently at home to help her control her weight.

You may feel your only choices are

- Pull her aside and ask her to stop eating the chips and juice.
- Keep quiet until you are headed home and then express your annoyance about how much she ate at the party.
- Say nothing but make sure you tighten up the snacking even more at home.
- Ignore the whole thing and hope tomorrow will be a better day.

Here is a tip to avoid this situation: Before the party, take your teen aside and acknowledge that social situations are difficult ones when anyone is trying to manage their eating and ask her how she thinks she could handle the situation. Listen and work from what she says. If she needs help thinking of strategies, you could suggest

- Planning the time she will visit the buffet and going only once.
- Trying to fill her plate half full of salad, vegetables, or fruit.

- Staying with one helping of ice cream and cake.
- Picking up sparkling water to carry with her to have something in her hands while others are snacking.
- Offering to bring a dish or appetizer to the party and making it a healthy one so your teen has some options. Suggest that your teen make it.
- Agreeing to talk after the party and debrief to see how the strategies she used worked. This is a chance to have a compassionate conversation and a learning opportunity.
- Planning what she can do the next time she finds herself in this situation.

Key Points to Remember

 Your adolescent is increasing her independence, but you are still her most important support. Keep the lines of communication open and ask your teen's pediatrician for help if needed.

 Skills like goal setting, taking small steps toward success, and understanding setbacks not only are important for managing weight but are life skills as well.

 Involving your teen in meal planning and cooking can be a shared effort that builds skills, encourages creativity, and makes a real contribution to family life.

 Changes in mood, behavior, communication, activity level, sleep, and other routines can indicate a problem with bullying, depression, anxiety, or other risky behavior. If you are worried, ask your teen's pediatrician for help.

Resources

Bleich SN, Wolfson JA. Trends in SSBs and snack consumption among children by age, body weight, and race/ethnicity. *Obesity (Silver Spring).* 2015;23(5):1039–1046

Frankowski BL, Leader IC, Duncan PM. Strength-based interviewing. *Adolesc Med State Art Rev.* 2009;20(1):22–40

Golden NH, Schneider M, Wood C; American Academy of Pediatrics Committee on Nutrition, Committee on Adolescence, Section on Obesity. Preventing obesity and eating disorders in adolescents. *Pediatrics.* 2016;138(3):e20161649

Lifshitz F. Obesity in children. *J Clin Res Pediatr Endocrinol.* 2008;1(2):53–60

Lyerly JE, Huber LR, Warren-Findlow J, Racine EF, Dmochowski J. Is breakfast skipping associated with physical activity among U.S. adolescents? A cross-sectional study of adolescents aged 12-19 years, National Health and Nutrition Examination Survey (NHANES). *Public Health Nutr.* 2014;17(4):896–905

Pearson N, Biddle SJ, Gorely T. Family correlates of fruit and vegetable consumption in children and adolescents: a systematic review. *Public Health Nutr.* 2009;12(2):267–283

Chapter 13

When Challenges Arise

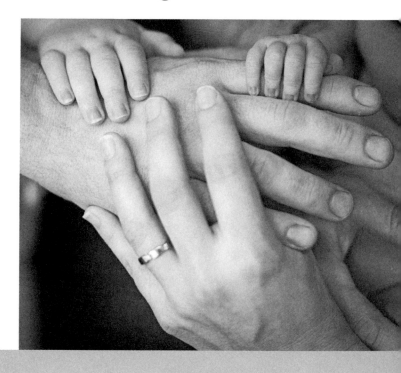

If you've ever tried to lose a few excess pounds yourself, you know that the journey toward weight loss is filled with challenges. It's no different when your child walks along that same path toward a healthier life. No matter how conscientious you and your child are, problems will arise and obstacles will surface. In this chapter, we'll describe some common hurdles—and solutions—that you might have already confronted or could encounter in the weeks and months ahead.

When you are actively working on helping your child achieve a healthy weight, there are natural questions that come up about family routines, your child's behavior, and the pros and cons of making a change. These kinds of questions are part of the normal process of making changes in a family's lifestyle, so don't hesitate to discuss your thoughts with your child's pediatrician. Here are some examples of common questions parents ask.

"I'd like to give my kids more fruits and vegetables, but fresh produce is too expensive!" Fresh fruits and vegetables are an investment in a healthier lifestyle. Unfortunately, it can also seem as if you are making an investment decision to buy them. Some parents worry about the cost of fresh produce, but they also worry about preparation time or are afraid of seeing fruits and vegetables spoil or go uneaten. Fresh fruits and vegetables may be more affordable than you think. Particularly if you buy them when they're in season, they'll be much more reasonably priced than at other times of the year. Also, compare the costs of produce to other foods that you may already be buying for your child. For example, processed foods—from cookies to potato chips—are not only more expensive, but they certainly aren't as nutritious as fresh fruits and vegetables.

A number of studies have shown that it may be feasible for most families to add fruits and vegetables to their food shopping. The US Department of Agriculture analyzed and released data from household food purchases made in 1999, including multiple types of fruits and vegetables. The researchers concluded that the average American can purchase 4 servings of vegetables and 3 servings of fruits for just 64 cents a day. If this figure were adjusted to today's costs, the price might be an average of less than a dollar a day. No matter how you analyze the numbers, that's a great deal. The same study found that two-thirds of all fresh fruits and more than half of all fresh vegetables are less costly than processed versions of the same produce. Additionally, frozen and canned fruits and vegetables are just as nutritious as their fresh counterparts and often are less expensive.

Learning to cook fruits and vegetables can add a variety of tastes and textures to meals and allow cooked versions to be frozen for later. For example, if you got a great deal on carrots at the store, cook enough for your meal and add extra to freeze for when vegetables are at a premium price.

To avoid wasting food, it is important to help your family incorporate fruits and vegetables into its routine. Cutting up fruits and putting them on the plate with the meal, trying a new "vegetable of the week," and planting some lettuce or tomatoes with your child are some ways to work produce into family menu. Here are some additional ideas.

- Pair a new vegetable with one your child likes and model how much you are enjoying eating both.
- Have your older child help prepare a vegetable dish with you for the family.
- Place fruit slices in water and keep a pitcher in the refrigerator for a colorful and healthy drink.
- A mixture of cut-up fruit makes a great dessert.

- Try a new vegetable dish from a different culture or one you remember from your childhood.
- Leave some fruits or vegetables on the counter so they are easily accessible. Your child may be more tempted to grab these to eat when they are in plain view.

"I'd prefer to feed a variety of vegetables to my child, but he absolutely hates vegetables. The only 'vegetables' he'll eat are French fries. That's it!"
Sometimes it can seem as if all you do is nag at your child to "finish his vegetables." How do you get the job done without feeling like all you talk about is food? As a parent, your job is to provide your child with well-balanced meals, including a variety of vegetables. Once the food is on the plate in front of him, he may choose whether to eat it. Sure, it can be frustrating when kids push the plate away and refuse to even try something new, but be persistent. The good news is that, over time, most children will develop a taste for enough healthy foods—even some vegetables—to be eating a balanced diet.

Some children may be more agreeable to consuming vegetables if you ask them to help you in the kitchen while you're preparing meals. They may be more receptive if you add vegetables to a pasta dish or put them in soups or meat loaf. For older children, a good snack might be cherry tomatoes or cut-up vegetables with yogurt dip if they prefer raw rather than cooked vegetables. When eating in restaurants, accompany children on trips through the salad bar; expose them to vegetables they may never have tried at home.

Meanwhile, continue to serve as a role model. If your child sees you eating vegetables, he's more likely to try them. Have him get used to the idea that vegetables are part of every lunch and dinner and can make great snacks. Remember that your child will need to have at least 1 serving of fruits and vegetables with every meal and snack to meet the recommended 5 servings a day.

"I know my child shouldn't have dessert with dinner every night or sweetened juices whenever he wants them, but I feel terrible if he complains about feeling deprived." It is hard to hear your child say "it's not fair," and children have a way of making us lose sight of why we're making healthy dietary changes. As a parent, your child's health is your top priority, and that may require making some adjustments in what he eats and the amount of physical activity he gets.

Of course, you don't want your child to feel deprived, and there's no need for you to eliminate his favorite desserts from his life. However, save those high-calorie foods, like rich ice cream or chocolate chip cookies, for special occasions and serve appropriate portion sizes when you do. At the same time, introduce him to healthier desserts, such as a dish of strawberries or a piece of angel food cake. When beverages are concerned, rely more often on low-fat milk or water rather than sugar-laden soft drinks or juices. Before long, he'll stop demanding the high-calorie, high-fat treats that he once craved.

"I'm willing to get unhealthy foods out of the house, but other adults in the home haven't come on board yet. They tell me that they've been drinking sugary soft drinks all their lives and they're not willing to give them up." Getting family members on board can feel like you are pushing uphill, but it is important to create the healthiest possible environment for your child. To be realistic, most family members could use some help with healthy eating and activity themselves. If other adults in the home insist on keeping high-fat snacks or high-calorie drinks in the cupboard or refrigerator, those kinds of temptations aren't fair to your child. To support your child's efforts to lose weight, it's essential for the entire family to get involved. The family needs to sit down and discuss the implications of continuing to live a lifestyle of poor eating choices. If the others still can't be convinced of the potential consequences of doing their own things, perhaps your child's pediatrician can talk with them. With your child's health at stake, your pediatrician may be able to motivate the others to give some ground. If they need to have sugary soft drinks, ask them to limit them to school or work and leave those kinds of snacks out of the house.

"My own mother seems to understand how important it is for my child to lose weight, but she still thinks it's a grandmother's prerogative to give my child candy whenever we visit. How can I convince her to get rid of that candy dish?" Grandparents are special people in our children's lives. They want to be loved by their grandchildren more than anything in the world, and giving them some of the sugary snacks they like can seem like one way to make them happy. When you talk with your child's grandmother or grandfather, you need to emphasize that your child's health comes first and point out the health risks your child faces unless he eats more nutritiously, one meal and one snack after another. As accustomed as Grandma may be to baking cookies when the grandchildren visit, you can probably appeal to her strong desire to give your child the best possible chance of living a healthy life. You can also help to find ways for grandparents to treat their grandchildren without using food. Here are some ways they can do that.

- Bring a special book with them that they can read to your child.
- Cook their favorite healthy dish with their grandchild.
- Have family story and playtime.
- Take a walk together or go to the park.
- Go to the local county fair or the zoo.

"I realize that when the family goes out to dinner, we should stay away from fast-food restaurants most of the time, but whenever we drive by one of those places, my child pleads with me to stop." It's fine to eat at fast-food restaurants once in a while. Because of their high-calorie fare, though, don't make it a habit.

When you visit these types of restaurants, order carefully for the family, finding choices to keep your child happy without sabotaging his healthier eating efforts. Whenever possible, for example, select a grilled chicken sandwich without any dressing for your child. If he insists on a hamburger, choose the smaller size, not the supersized double burger. Order a salad with low-fat dressing that he can eat as part of his meal.

Rather than over-relying on fast-food restaurants, choose to eat at sit-down family restaurants more frequently and look for healthy options on the menu. Split a dinner between the two of you. You will save money and eat healthier!

"Snacking before bedtime may not be a good idea for my child while he's trying to lose weight, but when I was growing up, my mother always gave us cookies and milk before we went to bed. It's just something that I feel comfortable doing, and it would be hard to do things differently." There is nothing inherently wrong with a bedtime snack, but you are focused on keeping your child at a healthy weight and may need to adjust the kinds of snacks you're offering.

In general, try to limit the number of snacks to 2 per day. For those late-night munchies, make choices that contribute to overall healthy eating. Snack time is an ideal time to add to your child's intake of fruits and vegetables or offer a glass of milk. If you implement this at the onset of bedtime snacking, your child will know that if he is hungry, the only option is a piece of fruit or nothing at all.

Also, think about what else was special about your bedtime routine as a child, or how you want to make your child's bedtime routine a special time just to be together, such as reading a book or singing. This can help take the emphasis off having to have a food treat.

"I understand that healthy eating is the best way for my child to lose weight, but I sometimes think that he could benefit from a little kick-start, and the latest fad diets promise fast results. What's wrong with following one of these diets for a few weeks to get him off to a good start?" Most people have lost weight at some point in their lives—but then gained it all back. They know that fad diets don't work, at least over the long term, but the alluring promises on magazine covers and television (TV) are often too tempting to resist.

Unfortunately, fad diets can be dangerous. They often emphasize a single food or food group, and they can be particularly risky for growing children for whom balanced nutrition is extremely important.

As we've emphasized throughout this book, you need to put your child's health and well-being first. Don't be persuaded by promises of overnight weight loss. Instead, stick with a plan for good nutrition and physical activity like the one described in these pages. Your child's weight loss will be gradual and safe and have the best chance for permanent success.

"I feel that I can control what my child eats at home, but when he's at child care, I have no control over what the child care provider gives him. He's served whatever the other kids eat." Express your concerns to the child care staff. Even if the facility serves identical meals to all the children, make some suggestions for fine-tuning the menu in the direction of healthier foods. The staff may turn out to be much more flexible than you expected and might be willing to bend to your requests, perhaps serving your youngster a turkey sandwich and small salad for lunch instead of a hamburger and French fries. Most child care centers today offer healthier menu options to promote healthier eating, such as a fruit with every meal, a veggie at lunch, and a veggie at snack time, such as cucumber slices with pitas and hummus. Parents should receive a menu handout for each month so they are aware of the meals being served each day.

If you're sensing some reluctance on their part, offer to pack your child's lunch and/or snacks for school to make sure that he's eating foods supportive of the family's commitment to more nutritious eating. Many child care centers have allergy restrictions and may not allow parents to pack their own child's lunch, so talk with the workers to create options that work best with your child.

"I'd love to sign my child up for a fitness program, but we just can't afford it."
Kids can enjoy the benefits of physical activity without busting the family
budget. Play is the major way kids can increase their activity. You don't
need costly exercise equipment like treadmills, nor do you have to enroll
them in classes with expensive sign-up fees. Outdoor play in a safe area
can be a major help to increasing physical activity. Plan to get together on
the weekend with school or neighborhood friends and plan fun indoor/
outdoor activities to get the kids moving. Often, local gyms offer open
gym time for kids to run around and use equipment suitable for their
age. Local pools are often inexpensive and can be a fun family outing.

Walking is one of the best forms of exercise, and it doesn't require any
special equipment, other than a good pair of walking shoes. If the entire
family gets involved, your child is more likely to be motivated to walk
regularly. In fact, the best forms of physical activity are family activities.
Keep them fun, and your child won't feel that he's missing out on the
formal program. Going to the park or on a bike ride will help keep your
child out of the house, get him active, and increase family time together.

**"Yes, my child knows that he needs to become more physically active, but
he has so much homework, plus piano lessons after school, and there's just
no time for exercise."** So many of today's kids lead very busy lives. It
seems as though their planned activities start immediately after school
and continue until well after nightfall. If you think about it, there's
probably sometime in your child's afternoon and evening, even just
15 or 20 minutes, when he could fit in some physical activity.

Remember, activity needs to become a *priority* in your child's life. That
means that exercise wins out over video games or watching TV every
time. After school, he can play catch with the neighborhood kids in the
park down the block or play a game of hoops on the driveway. Frankly,
there aren't too many kids who don't have a few minutes to spare each day
for squeezing in some physical activity. Physical activity promotes motor
and mental development and is essential for developing coordination.

"My child should be getting more physical activity, but in our neighborhood, I don't think it's safe for him to be playing outdoors." Safety concerns are important, but don't let them keep your child sedentary. There are plenty of ways for him to stay active other than playing in your front yard or on the neighborhood playground. He can participate in a local or community swimming program or join a karate class. He can stay active indoors at home by dancing to his favorite music, spinning a hula hoop, jumping rope, or doing chores like straightening up his room. You can plan a family activity or bike ride on the weekends and take him on errands with you where there is an opportunity to increase his walking.

"Eating right and being active makes sense, but my teenager has so much weight to lose that we've been talking about weight-loss surgery. Is that something we should consider?" Although the overwhelming majority of weight-loss surgeries are being performed in adults, a relatively small number of teenagers have undergone the procedure. However, this is *major* surgery, and the decision to have the operation should not be made hastily.

Weight-loss surgery is only advisable for adolescents with severe obesity for whom more conservative weight-loss measures haven't worked, particularly if they also have developed serious obesity-related medical conditions, such as high blood pressure, diabetes, and sleep apnea.

Your pediatrician can provide an initial assessment of whether your teenager might be a candidate for surgery. If the pediatrician refers you for a consultation to a weight-loss program that performs these procedures, you and your adolescent will meet with the surgeon and the pediatrician as well as a number of other specialists, including clinical psychologists and nutritionists. You and your teenager will have the opportunity to discuss the potential benefits of the operation, plus get your questions answered about the complications sometimes associated with the operation, like infections, bleeding, and blood clots. Most programs are very careful about proper preparation of patients for surgery, allowing enough time for parents and adolescents to understand the benefits, complications, and permanent changes in lifestyle that surgery entails.

"How much weight should my child lose? Will he ever be at a normal weight?"
An elevated body mass index is a marker for excess weight that can
compromise your child's health and well-being. If he already has some
of the comorbidities of obesity, like elevated lipids or sleep apnea, the
first step is addressing his current health problems. This includes getting
his lipids back into the typical range and treating his sleep apnea at
the same time you are working to help him stop his weight gain by
improving his nutrition and sleep, increasing physical activity, and
reducing sedentary time. The next step is to aim for gradual weight loss
by consistent lifestyle change. Even loss of 10% of his weight can bring
his obesity-related comorbidities back toward normal. Even with a
perfect lifestyle, our genetics will play a role in our bodies' ultimate
height and weight, but the goal is to achieve the healthiest lifestyle
possible and the healthiest weight possible. Each child is unique, and
your child's pediatrician can help set your child's individual weight
loss goals to minimize the negative health effects of obesity and
promote lifelong health.

Key Points to Remember

 Setbacks are perfectly normal and happen to everyone on the
way to achieving a goal.

It is important to try to understand why your child and family
got derailed from the healthy goal you set and to find a way
to address what is getting in the way. This makes it a learning
experience for everyone.

 Enlisting all family members in troubleshooting can turn up
some unexpected ideas on how to move forward and helps
get everyone on the same team.

Encourage adolescents to take responsibility of some aspect
of their health care.

Afterword

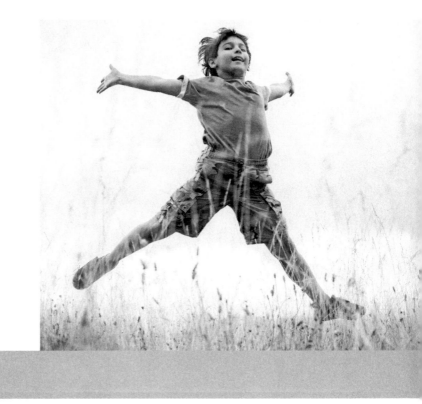

Now that you have read *Achieving a Healthy Weight for Your Child,* I hope you have been able to try some of the ideas for healthier living suggested in this book and have been encouraged and inspired that your child and family can achieve a healthier lifestyle. Working toward a healthy weight is a process with accomplishments along the way that can make the whole family proud and give your child the confidence to achieve the goals she sets. Being able to help your child overcome setbacks and transition her to making healthy lifestyle decisions as an adult is a proud accomplishment for any parent. As a parent, you are not in this alone. Your child's pediatrician, extended family, school, and community are all resources to assist you in helping your child on this journey. Being a parent of a child struggling with weight can be challenging but rewarding too, as you guide your child to better health.

Goals for the Future

As you, your family, and your child move ahead on a journey toward better health and achieving a healthy weight, there are a couple of tips that will help keep you on the right track.

Understanding Weight Goals
In some cases, particularly if your child is younger and still growing, your child's pediatrician may recommend that your child not lose any additional weight but, rather, maintain her present weight until her

height catches up. As she becomes taller, her body mass index (BMI) will improve as her weight stays the same. By contrast, the goals for a teenager may be different. If your adolescent has already reached her full height, the only way to lower her BMI is to reduce her weight, and this may start by helping her keep her current weight stable and moving on to slow and steady weight loss supervised by her pediatrician. But, as you have read, weight should not be her only goal. In fact, success is achieving lifelong habits that will help her improve her health now and as an adult.

Health Goals

As you read in Chapter 1, obesity contributes to many serious health problems. Your pediatrician will help identify the specific health risks faced by your child and help you, your family, and your child set goals for improving her overall health.

To reach these goals, you and your child should continue to place an emphasis on a healthy lifestyle, including

- Striving for healthy nutrition
- Increasing daily physical activity
- Reducing the time spent in front of screens
- Getting adequate sleep

Lifestyle modifications like these should become you and your child's day-to-day goals, beginning in the short term and then lasting a life-time. Having the support of the entire family is the best way to ensure that these new healthy habits will become a routine. The key is to turn these lifestyle improvements into your family's new normal. In earlier times, perhaps it was normal for your child to drink 3 sugary soft drinks a day; now, her new normal is to drink water or low-fat milk instead. She's not on a diet—she just has a new normal way of living.

What if Your Child Backslides?

No one's perfect. Everyone slips up from time to time. In adopting the family's new nutritional and active lifestyle, your child may do just fine for weeks, but then she might respond to the stress of final examinations by sneaking food or making inappropriate choices in the school cafeteria. During the holidays, she might overindulge in the traditional desserts that Grandma makes. If the entire family has a particularly busy week, all of you may eat out more than usual, and regular physical activity may be sacrificed.

When you're talking about adopting a healthy lifestyle over the long term, these kinds of occasional lapses are inevitable. No matter what the reason, when you notice that your child is backsliding, the key is to help her get back on track as soon as possible. Don't allow the slip to turn into a long, downhill slide. Encourage your child so she doesn't become bogged down by frustration or disappointment. In fact, the sooner you intervene, the better her chances are of bouncing back, barely missing a beat. Don't forget to remove easy temptations, such as unhealthy snacks and sugary drinks.

How can you minimize the risk of future backsliding? Spend some time with your child and think about why the problem occurred. Was the lapse an indication that your child has started making poor choices? Did some short-term distractions take place that could recur? Once you and your child understand the reasons that she stumbled, they're less likely to happen again.

In the meantime, rather than becoming preoccupied with a setback, keep your child focused on everything that she has done right over the past few weeks and months. Remind her of the progress she's made, and encourage her to keep moving forward. Let her know that despite the backsliding, she's still headed in the right direction.

PREPARING PLAN B

When you least expect it, life events can intervene and derail all your and your child's efforts toward a healthier life. Perhaps Dad goes into the hospital for surgery; Mom decides to go back to school 3 nights a week while also keeping her job during the day; Grandma becomes ill, throwing everyone's schedule awry; or you're moving from one house to another, disrupting your usual routines for a couple weeks or more.

However, backsliding during these times can often be avoided if you and your family plan in advance for any events that could sabotage your child's progress toward a healthier life. If you know that a family member's surgery is on the horizon, for example, why not have a fallback plan—plan B—already in place? Rather than letting events that lead to abandoning health-supporting lifestyle changes roll over you, why not decide as a family ahead of time how you're going to deal with them? What steps have worked in the past when disruptions occurred (for example, keeping meals simple and preparing and freezing them ahead of time), and can you implement them again in the future?

Stressful, unexpected events are a part of life, and you need to make sure that they don't undermine the progress your child has already made.

Looking Ahead

Success in achieving a healthy weight isn't going to happen overnight. It's a process, and you should approach it one step at a time. Even when the long-term goals seem challenging, you can and should celebrate the small achievements, one day after another. As your child makes changes in her nutrition and physical activity, they will contribute to her overall success, and you should offer praise for every one of these advances, one week after the next.

Along the way, stay in touch with your child's pediatrician. The doctor can help you answer the question, "How are we doing?" by monitoring your child's weight and the health improvements that are taking place. Your pediatrician also can assist your family in rising above any setbacks. Consider your child's pediatrician a partner throughout this process.

As you continue to implement the lifestyle strategies described in this book, you should be pleased with the progress your child is making. Remember, you have taken an important step to help your child achieve better lifelong health.

Appendix

The Pediatrician's Role at a Glance

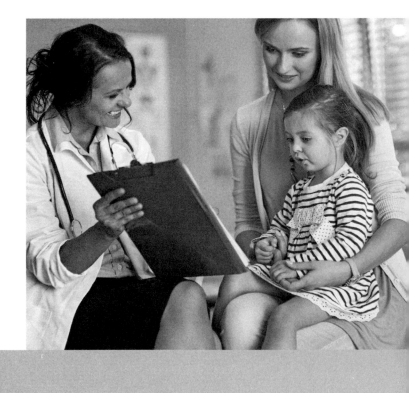

Before starting any type of weight program, it is important to discuss your child's weight with your child's pediatrician. This book provides the support and guidance you need for your child to achieve a healthy weight. Several chapters outline the integral role the pediatrician plays in this lifestyle change. Here are some of the various ways your child's pediatrician can help, collected from chapters in this book.

Talking With Your Child's Pediatrician (From Chapter 3)

Before your child moves from a sedentary to a more active way of life, and particularly if he has any health problems, talk with your child's pediatrician. Your pediatrician will be able to tell you how to ensure that exercising is a safe and enjoyable experience for your child. Above all, ask the pediatrician whether your child has any physical limitations or any accommodations that are needed to participate or allow regular activity that you need to keep in mind. For example, many parents think that children who have asthma can't play outdoors on a cold day, or they'll risk having asthmatic episodes. Your pediatrician can help you and your child plan for safe outdoor activity by including this option in your child's asthma plan. Children with special health care needs are often more at risk for obesity and need to be physically active. Check with your pediatrician for community opportunities for activities geared to your child and recommendations for activities to be included in your child's individualized education program (IEP) for school.

Partnering With Your Child's Pediatrician (From Chapter 4)

Since the time your child was born, you have relied on her pediatrician to play multiple roles in your child's life, from providing physical examinations to treating her illnesses to administering her immunizations on schedule. Don't overlook the important supportive role your pediatrician can play by partnering with your family in helping your child achieve a healthy weight.

Each time you visit the pediatrician's office, particularly for scheduled checkups, your doctor or a nurse will weigh and measure your child and calculate her body mass index. He or she will check your child's overall health status and monitor any obesity-related health conditions she may have, such as high blood pressure or high cholesterol levels.

Your pediatrician can also talk with your child about her weight problem at a level appropriate for her age. The doctor can help you and your child prioritize the changes that need to be made first to get her weight under control and help you set some health goals, including lifestyle changes such as eating more healthfully, becoming more physically active, and watching less TV.

Also, turn to your child's pediatrician for guidance on child development issues. The doctor can answer questions like, "At my child's age, what is she capable of doing on her own as we're adopting a more healthful lifestyle?" As you might guess, and your pediatrician can help explain, a 14-year-old is able to do much more than a 4-year-old. It isn't developmentally appropriate, for example, to put your 4-year-old in charge of getting her own snacks from the refrigerator and expect her to make appropriate choices, but a 14-year-old who you've educated about healthy snacking might be trusted to do so.

Selecting a Pediatrician (From Chapter 7)

Choosing a pediatrician is an important decision that you should make before your baby is born. Once your newborn arrives, it will be comforting to know that you have a pediatrician available who can care for your baby from birth, give him his very first examination, and answer all your questions.

New parents sometimes interview several pediatricians before making their choice. These interviews can usually be arranged during the last few months of your pregnancy. If you need the names of a few pediatricians, you can ask your obstetrician and check the American Academy of Pediatrics HealthyChildren.org Web site under "Find a Pediatrician." You can also ask friends and family members with children about the pediatricians they use and whether they're happy with their choice. You want to select a pediatrician who you feel you can talk to.

During your interviews with the pediatrician, ask questions like

- "How soon after birth will you see my baby for his first examination?"
- "At what intervals do you recommend seeing newborns for healthy baby visits?"
- "Are you willing to respond to questions by telephone, text, or e-mail?"
- "When you're unavailable, what pediatrician will I be able to reach instead?"
- "What procedures do you advise in case of an emergency?"
- "What are the fees for the health care services you provide, and do you accept the insurance my family has?"

Many additional topics discussed in this chapter and throughout the book can be raised during your interviews and subsequent visits to the pediatrician's office, including the benefits of breastfeeding and the prevention and management of obesity in children.

The Pediatrician's Role (From Chapter 8)

To make sure your baby is growing well, your pediatrician will measure your baby's length and weight and then plot these measurements on the grow curve (figures 8-1–8-4). A measurement called *weight for length* can tell you and your pediatrician if your baby's weight is growing faster than her height; if so, your pediatrician will monitor your baby's feeding and activity.

The Pediatrician's Role (From Chapter 9)

By now you know that your pediatrician won't rely solely on visual observation to determine whether your child's weight is at a healthy level. The most reliable guide is where your child's height, weight, and weight for length (for children younger than 2 years) fall on a standard growth chart. If the chart shows that your toddler is a little heavier than typical, your pediatrician can help you determine what actions are most appropriate at this age. As a general rule, however, you should never restrict calories in a toddler without the guidance of your pediatrician because you don't want to risk interfering with his normal growth and development. In evaluating his increase in weight, your pediatrician will ask about any signs or symptoms you've seen in your child and perform a physical examination to make sure he doesn't have any health problems that could be causing the weight gain.

The next thing is to see what could be causing him to gain weight more rapidly. Here is where the detective work begins. For most children, the proper health-promoting strategies are not complicated. They involve guidance that you've heard before.

- Optimize your child's nutrition.
- Make sure he gets plenty of physical activity and minimize screen time.
- Make sure he gets enough sleep.

An Action Step: Record Keeping

One of the most helpful things you can do as you try to unravel your child's weight gain is to keep a record of everything he eats and his physical activity, screen time habits, and sleep behavior. This means that everyone caring for your child needs to keep track of what they are feeding him and what his sleep and activity schedule is like. This isn't as hard as it sounds because you are writing down the daily routines as you go. In general, 3 days of records, including the weekends, is enough to start to see patterns that are getting in the way of healthy eating, activity, and sleeping. You'll need to put in the amount and what kind of food your child ate or drank, wake-up and bedtime, length of nap time, and how much screen and playtime. Use Table 9-1 to record the information you've collected, or copy this template into a journal. If your child is with Grandma or in child care, ask if they can add to the record. You may be surprised at just how much is going on in your child's day!

Table 9-1. My Child's Daily Routine			
	Thursday	**Friday**	**Saturday**
Wake-up time Breakfast Screen time Snack Active play			
Lunch Nap Screen time Snack Active play			
Dinner Active play Screen time Bedtime			

The Pediatrician's Role (From Chapter 10)

The preschool years are a time when a growing number of children are first identified as having an elevated BMI. If your child has a BMI above the 85th percentile, your child's pediatrician will do 3 things.

Obtain a Growth History

Your pediatrician will look at your child's growth over time to see when her weight began to increase faster than her height and her BMI began increasing. This gives your doctor a picture of when there might have been a change in your child's lifestyle or health that resulted in increased weight gain (or decreased height growth). Knowing this time frame can often provide clues to help get your child back on track to a healthy weight.

Medical Evaluation

Your pediatrician will review a detailed history of your child's health to make sure that she doesn't have any rare health condition that could cause extra weight gain or health problems caused by her extra weight gain. Your doctor will also review her medications and ask about family history, focusing on any obesity-related chronic health conditions. Along with this, your pediatrician will perform a physical examination. Your pediatrician may also order specific laboratory tests as part of the medical evaluation.

Nutrition and Activity Assessment

Your pediatrician will ask specific questions about diet, physical activity, and lifestyle to get a picture of your child's daily eating and activity routines.

The Pediatrician's Role (From Chapter 11)

During your child's school-age years, he may see your pediatrician for routine well-child examinations about every 1 to 2 years. If your child has obesity, you may need to schedule appointments more often. Your pediatrician can regularly calculate his BMI and help guide your family toward better nutrition and more physical activity as well as help you troubleshoot if your child is having difficulties in one health-related area or another.

If your child has a BMI greater than the 95th percentile, your pediatrician may do 3 things.

1 **Your pediatrician will ask a series of questions to find out if your child has been affected by any obesity-related health conditions.** These are medical problems that result from the effect of obesity on other body systems, such as the lungs, heart, liver, and bones. Your pediatrician may ask about headaches, vision problems, difficulty breathing normally or with exercise, stomach problems, constipation, urination, and pain or discomfort with your child's joints, especially his hips and knees. Your pediatrician will also ask about your child's mood, feelings, and depression and if he has been bullied or teased. Your pediatrician will perform a physical examination. It is important for your child's well-being that your pediatrician understands your child's health status as completely as possible. If necessary, your pediatrician will order laboratory studies based on your child's history and the physical examination.

2 **Your pediatrician will want to know as much detail as possible about your child's lifestyle, family eating and activity patterns, and family and cultural traditions that affect nutrition and activity.** (See the diet and activity record in Table 9-1.) Treatment of obesity in children starts with taking a close look at what they are eating and what kind of activity and inactivity they engage in every day, as well as understanding their sleep patterns.

❸ Instilling change is challenging, and your pediatrician may use something called motivational interviewing to help you identify the goals you have for your child. Motivational interviewing is a way of having a conversation that allows you to focus on what is most important to you and your child and helps you and your child pick which changes you feel most motivated to tackle.

The next sections will give you some ideas of an approach to healthy eating and activity to help you pick a starting place for your child for a healthy lifestyle change.

The Pediatrician's Role (From Chapter 12)

How Your Teen's Pediatrician Can Help

- **Encourage the conversation.** Sometimes teens do not want to talk about their weight. It can be an uncomfortable topic for them, and they may not open up quickly—or at all. If you are having trouble talking with your teen about her weight, your teen's pediatrician can help get the ball rolling. If it is time for a checkup, your pediatrician will be discussing height, weight, and body mass index (BMI) just like your pediatrician has been doing all along, opening the door to talk with your teen about her health choices.
- Don't be surprised if the conversation starts to be aimed at your teen. Watch and see how this goes. Many times you can use this as a jumping-off point for continuing the discussion at home.
- If you become concerned and want to talk about your teen's weight between well checkups, you can always schedule a visit with your teen's pediatrician to do just that. Just be sure you and your teen have discussed the reason for the visit before you both get to the appointment. If you want to talk by phone with your pediatrician beyond scheduling a visit, it is preferable to include your teen on the call. The message here is that you are in this together.

- **Evaluate her health and behaviors.** Adolescence is a crucial time to set the stage for the independence of young adulthood. Your pediatrician will evaluate your teen for obesity-related conditions and risky health behaviors. They may want to do this in private, and that can be an important step in the transition to your adolescent's self-care. However, also having a family-based discussion is critical to setting attainable nutrition and activity goals and making sure the family can provide needed support and all be on the same page.

- **Assess the environment.** Peers, school, and the neighborhood can all be powerful influences over your adolescent's health behaviors. Your pediatrician will want to understand what is happening in the environment that surrounds your adolescent. The pediatrician may want to discuss these external factors in private, as well.

- **Assess and understand your adolescent's mood and mental health.** Adolescence can be a time of increased stress, escalated expectations, and increased body consciousness. Adding obesity to the mix can often result in difficulties with anxiety, self-esteem, or depression. It is important for your teen's pediatrician to understand just how your adolescent is thinking and feeling and be able to offer support and treatment if needed.

Index

Index